Conflict, Culture and Identity in GP Training

Jennifer L. Johnston

Conflict, Culture and Identity in GP Training

palgrave
macmillan

Jennifer L. Johnston
Centre for Medical Education
Queen's University Belfast
Belfast, UK

ISBN 978-981-19-2963-2   ISBN 978-981-19-2964-9   (eBook)
https://doi.org/10.1007/978-981-19-2964-9

Cover pattern © John Rawsterne/patternhead.com

This Palgrave Pivot imprint is published by the registered company Springer Nature Singapore Pte Ltd.
The registered company address is: 152 Beach Road, #21-01/04 Gateway East, Singapore 189721, Singapore

Problematising structures of GP training in the UK, this innovative approach combines empirical and theoretical scholarship in examining the experiences of GP trainees working in hospitals. Drawing on trainee narratives and privileging the analysis of social language-in-use, Johnston describes primary care medicine as a separate paradigm with its own philosophy, identity and practice. Casting primary care as in longstanding conflict with secondary care, the lower status of primary care in the world of medicine is explored, along with significant identity challenges for GP trainees positioned at the coalface of conflict. As a result, radical changes to the structures of GP training are proposed.

Jennifer Johnston is a Clinical Reader at Queen's University Belfast, and a critical educationalist. She is a practising GP in a part of Belfast, Northern Ireland, with high socioeconomic deprivation and believes in education as a vehicle for social change in healthcare. This book has been developed from her original PhD work, which won the Association for the Study of Medical Education Best Original Research Paper in 2016.

For my family

CONTENTS

CHAPTER 1

Introduction

Abstract This chapter introduces the questions explored throughout the text and sets its social, cultural and historical contexts, including the structures of GP training and the development of power dynamics in the socialised UK National Health Service (NHS). Aimed at a key audience of GP educators and clinical academics, a sociocultural conceptual framework used is outlined in a way which is approachable to those previously unfamiliar with social theory. Brief methodological details for the empirical elements are also described.

Keywords GP • Identity • Medical education • Sociocultural theory

This book is intended for medical educators and anyone involved in training general practitioners (GPs), including GP and hospital supervisors. At the heart of the book are two empirical research projects: one in which seven new GP trainees, based in hospital posts, tell their stories; and one in which another GP trainee narrates her story as she moves across hospital posts and into the community. These are important narratives, which highlight the difficulties and professional challenges to their identities faced by these doctors. They also give vital new insights into the broader discourses governing the relationship between general practice and hospital medicine, and the inequalities and power structures which result.

J. L. Johnston, *Conflict, Culture and Identity in GP Training*, https://doi.org/10.1007/978-981-19-2964-9_1

Throughout the book, a *critical sociocultural* framework is used to problematise the way in which new doctors become GPs. Language is used as a means to explore power dynamics and social actions, the most important of which for these purposes is identity development. Acknowledging that the field of medical education is diverse and that not all readers will be familiar with a sociological orientation, efforts are made to avoid jargon unless essential. Where it is necessary to use a jargon term this is followed by an explanation.

This introductory chapter outlines the theoretical framework around which the analyses are structured. This is simply a set of assumptions which taken together form a particular lens. Viewing the work through this lens allows some things to be foregrounded. Different lenses would, of course, likely give different results, making it essential to detail assumptions made at the very beginning. Methodological information for the two empirical chapters is also given in brief. The following two chapters present the empirical narratives, followed by two chapters in which these and other empirical literature are drawn together with theoretical perspectives. In the last chapter, radical changes to educational practice policy are suggested.

Finally, it is important to state at the outset that this is an emic (insider's) analysis; as the author, I am also a GP and medical educationalist. Approaching the work with reflexivity and humility, I hope it will resonate with other GPs, transfer to other primary care contexts, and spark interest in secondary care colleagues.

A NOTE ON TERMINOLOGY AND POSITIONING

In the UK National Health Service (NHS) on which this book centres, the term *primary care* is used to refer to community-based clinical generalism. Although secondary care clinics do take place in communities, they are specialty-focused, for example, community paediatrics. When the term *secondary care* is used here, it is used synonymously with specialist work, mainly taking place in hospital settings.

The primary research in Chaps. 2 and 3 is situated and not based on a statistical sample, meaning it is not generalisable in the same sense as biomedical research. Instead, the focus is on depth and meaning-making in keeping with a critical constructionist stance. This is a research philosophy common in social sciences and education, in which all data (and indeed all meaning) is considered to be *constructed* between people, rather than already there ready to be discovered. It is also an approach committed to problematising taken-for-granted knowledge, driven by an active social change agenda. In keeping with this orientation, concepts derived from non-generalisable data can be *transferrable* to other, similar contexts.

Examples of such contexts are likely to include other countries in the global north with developed healthcare systems. Similar divisions and tensions exist between community generalists and hospital specialists in such settings. Other terms used for GPs in these settings include *family doctor*, *family physician* and *primary care physician*.

SETTING THE SCENE

Since the NHS was founded, and even before, doctors have been serving their local communities as general medical practitioners. These family doctors embody the cradle-to grave-care for which the NHS was designed, offering longitudinal primary care to individuals and families on the basis of need alone. Based in surgeries often located in or near their own communities, GPs have the privilege of understanding context and the ability to develop therapeutic relationships with their patients over time. They stand as important patient advocates within the maelstrom of politically-influenced changes to the NHS.

GPs are, as their name suggests, clinical generalists, managing a huge array of conditions. Yet training schemes for general practice are the shortest of any in medicine, taking three years on average, and with as much as half that time spent working in specialised hospital environments [1]. New GPs are independent doctors long before their hospital peers, and are thrown into the rough and tumble of practice with various degrees of preparation for community-based primary care work [2].

Added to this, many trainees and qualified GPs experience stigma within the profession [3, 4]. This comes from hospital doctors and is directed at their career choice, the nature of their work, and a perceived lack of knowledge and skills relative to secondary care medics [5, 6]. This interesting power dynamic may not be particularly visible to the general public, who in general rate their GPs highly [7], but has a long social and cultural history [8]. While similar patterns can be seen across many Western countries [3], in the UK, the inequality between primary care (clinical generalists based in communities) and secondary care (clinical specialists based in hospitals and specialist clinics) is closely tied to the development of the NHS.

Although primary and secondary care doctors are closely and inevitably linked by the shared activity of patient care, the cultures and practices of each have developed along markedly different lines. Chapter 4 explores the idea of primary care as a separate *paradigm* of care, with its own philosophy, identity and practice. If primary care is one paradigm and secondary care another, then GP trainees working in hospitals are placed right at the interface between them. Studying their experiences offers a way in to understanding the longstanding tensions and misunderstanding between the two paradigms, and to explore the effects on GP trainees' professional development and identity.

WHY IDENTITIES ARE IMPORTANT

Identities are a central concept throughout the book. Broadly speaking, there are two broad streams of modern identity theory: a psychologically driven thread from Erikson's work, which focuses on individuals [9]; and a sociocultural thread from Goffman's work, which focuses on the relationships of individuals with societal and cultural groups [10]. The former considers identity as an integrative whole and as progressive over a lifetime. The latter, which is used here, emphasises the layers of relationships that people have with themselves, their social lives and activities, and their cultural surroundings. Identities (plural, not singular) are constructed through social interactions. They are changeable and never become truly fixed. Any one person can have lots of different identities, each of which may come into play depending on circumstances. These different identities may overlap or can even be in conflict with each other at times. For example, one commonly experienced identity conflict is the tension between being a parent and being at work. Most importantly, identities *mediate action* (facilitate the person to do things) [11]. This is why professional identities are important, because they mediate the activity taking place at work.

As social beings, it is the dialogue we have with others and the actions that we take across social, cultural, historical and political contexts which define who we are.

People engage in identity work every day through their regular activities. Using signs and symbols, either material or forms of language, are important ways of doing identity work [10]. Getting up and putting on clothes for work often signals an identity to others from a distance: for instance, a uniform for a soldier, a suit for a businessman, or scrubs for a surgeon. Particular props (*artefacts*) can be used to support identities:

respectively for the examples above, consider a gun, a briefcase and a scalpel, or a set or orders, a contract and a pre-surgical checklist.

As well as myriad smaller daily interactions, identities are also shaped by larger forces which provide an overarching influence. Some of the biggest are race, class and gender. Healthcare, like other social structures, is also subject to large-scale forms of power and influence, known as *discourses* [12]. For example, the UK NHS, a socialised form of healthcare inaugurated at a time of social progress just after the Second World War, was designed to offer healthcare for all which was free at the point of use. It was based on comprehensive public healthcare delivered according to need and not ability to pay. At the time of writing, however, the NHS has struggled for many years with underfunding and limitations to the service delivered [13]. This can be seen as a product of the prevailing economic discourse of *neoliberalism*, which prioritises free market forces and individualism in all sectors of public life [14]. Neoliberalism is also prevalent in tertiary (including medical) education, seen in the move of universities towards operating as competitive businesses, the monetisation of research and students as consumers [15].

Throughout this book, the major focus is on everyday social and cultural interactions which impact people's normal practices and therefore identities. There is no denying, however, the influence of 'big-D' (high level) discourses on these interactions, and so these are also explored in Chaps. 4 and 5.

MEDICAL TRAJECTORIES

Often, medical education is referred to as a continuum, implying a smooth transition across undergraduate and postgraduate training towards continuous professional development. This approach homogenises the wide variety of trainees at each level, their backgrounds and experiences, and glosses over any bumps they may encounter on the road to independent practice.

The basic structure of medical training is four to six years at university, followed by a mandatory two-year Foundation Programme and then entry into a specialist training Scheme [16]. Full registration with the regulator, the General Medical Council (GMC) is only granted at the end of the first year. A majority of placements are based in hospital, but it is possible to do a GP placement and some non-clinical placements are available, such as in academia. Most foundation rotations last four months each.

After completing the Foundation Programme satisfactorily, junior doctors are in a position to apply for specialty training. This lasts three years for general practice and five to eight years for secondary care specialties. In reality, though, many choose alternative routes at this time. The 2019 F2 Career Destinations Survey found only 46.4% of foundation doctors intended to go straight into training, many either taking a career break or working abroad for a year (colloquially known as the 'F3' year) [17]. According to the GMC, however, 90% of foundation programme leavers enter training schemes within three years [18].

While the UK government is planning for approximately 50% of medical graduates to become GPs, interest in GP careers has been reducing [19, 20]. In 2019, 31.6% of F2 leavers entering specialty training started a GP scheme, of which it was the first choice for 99.3% [17]. Along with poor retention, the cumulative effect has been a workforce crisis in general practice. The reasons for this are complex and related to high workload and burnout and poor job satisfaction [21]. From an educational perspective, early exposure to primary care and significant primary care experience are relevant to the recruitment of junior doctors into GP training [22, 23]. During medical school, most teaching takes place in hospital settings [24]. Given the relative paucity of primary care experience, foundation placements in general practice are an important initiative. Arguably, both future GPs and future hospital doctors can benefit from a better understanding of primary healthcare. The reasons behind the predominance of hospitals in undergraduate and early postgraduate training are historical and are discussed in later chapters.

Those wishing to become GPs, either directly or after time in a specialty training scheme, will apply to a regionally-organised GP training scheme. These were introduced in the 1980s as a means of improving the perception and professionalisation of GP training, which in the past had required no particular postgraduate training, with GPs learning entirely on the job. Schemes usually consist of eighteen months rotating around hospital specialties and eighteen months actually working in general practice [1]. GP trainees working in hospitals join the same rota as their specialty trainee peers, undertaking the same roles and responsibilities. This group therefore provide a significant service contribution to hospitals.

The workforce crisis in UK general practice is at risk of exacerbation from contemporary events such as Brexit (the UK's departure from the European Union) [25], politic rhetoric of a 'hostile environment' around immigration which may impact on international medical graduates (IMGs)

[26], and the impact of the 2020 coronavirus pandemic. Yet, the World Health Organisation identify strong primary healthcare as one of its most urgent health challenges for the 2020s [27]. Exploring conflict, culture and identity in general practice is an important way of defining challenges, supporting doctors in GP careers, and improving training processes.

IDENTITY CHALLENGES

Throughout this book, the complexities of training for general practice are treated as problematic in terms of identity. The structures of UK GP training reflect hegemonic (that is, dominant in a way which appears normal) assumptions about good education taking place in secondary care. This has been an accepted norm since Johns Hopkins School of Medicine integrated with its local hospital under William Osler in the 1890s [28]. Because of the structures of training, GP trainees face some specific challenges.

The length of GP training (the shortest available in the UK at three years) means that GPs move into the workplace as independent practitioners much earlier than their specialty training peers. Combined with relatively less exposure to general practice settings at undergraduate level, new GPs may not be well prepared for practice. Additionally, GPs, while often based in group surgeries, tend to work alone for most of the time with variable support available [29]. In response to the lack of support for new GPs, the Royal College of General Practitioners (RCGP) run a dedicated 'First 5' [years] programme of continuous professional development [30].

GP remains the only specialty training scheme where trainees spend half their training time working somewhere else. During the eighteen months based in hospital, trainees do the same job as specialty trainees with little or no attention paid to their final destination. Contact with the world of GP is often limited to a monthly day release programme. It is well documented that GP trainees may experience negativity from hospital doctors while in these posts. General practice may be misunderstood, perceived as 'secondary care light', or training seen as less different or easier to achieve. In the literature, negative experiences amongst hospital-based GP trainees ranges from well-intended misunderstanding of primary care work to open derision (the 'just a GP' syndrome) [5]. Longstanding misunderstanding and conflict between primary and secondary care plays out within the experiences of GP trainees in hospital placements. In narrating her own story of professional development, Giles comments on how her experience of negative attitudes to family medicine was a serious challenge during her residency [31]. In Beaulieu et al.'s qualitative study of trainees in Belgium, France and Canada, many had been told by hospital staff that they were "too bright" to become a GP [32]. Practically speaking, consultant supervisors who qualified before the foundation programme started in 2005 are unlikely to have had direct experience of working in primary care, whereas all trainees (and qualified GPs) will have had experience of hospital work. This may mean consultants are less aware of the differing training needs of GP trainees and hospital specialty trainees [33]. This situation has been worsened by the coronavirus pandemic from 2020 [34].

Furthermore, while frequent rotations are an accepted part of life for specialty trainees, GP trainees have the unique disadvantage of constantly moving between departments (for example, from acute medicine to paediatrics to psychiatry). This has a number of implications. Each hospital specialty has its own subculture and practice [35], the norms of which will need to be taken on board in addition to new content knowledge and clinical skills. A GP trainee who might have felt like a competent paediatric doctor yesterday is a complete newcomer to psychiatry. Unlike specialty trainees, growing expertise is not reflected in a progression in seniority, as it would be for a specialty trainee progressing through a training programme. For GP trainees, every new rotation means starting from scratch.

Structures and Contexts of General Practice

In this section, social, cultural and historical contexts of NHS general practice are outlined. Ways of being and relationships of power that have been developed over years have important contemporary effects. These strands of context are *dialogic* (in constant two-way dialogue [36]) with each other and with individuals, adding an extra layer of complexity.

Historical Development

The history of UK general practice is inextricably intertwined with the development of healthcare services in the UK, and with public health advances of the twentieth and twenty-first centuries.

Before the inception of the NHS in 1948, GPs worked in communities as private public health doctors. In 1911, the revolutionary National Insurance Act gave low-income workers (although not their families) access to sick pay and healthcare for the first time [37]. This was achieved through mandatory National Insurance payments, and GPs became contracted by local insurance committees to offer healthcare to this group. The background to the National Insurance Act was a Royal Commission into the state of public health in 1909 [38], showing a serious deficit in the care of poorer patients, although the more well-off were able to purchase general and specialist care. Tuberculosis was a serious public health problem. Following Germany's lead, then Chancellor of the Exchequer David Lloyd George introduced social insurance as an important means of improving national health.

Despite initial resistance, the scheme was eventually approved by British Medical Association (BMA) members. The BMA requested amendments to doctors' remuneration, representation and administration, as well as aspects of patient care. These included that the scheme should have an upper income limit excluding those able to pay for care, patients should have a free choice of doctor, and benefits should be administered by local health committees rather than friendly societies or insurance schemes. Having delayed implementation of the Act by a year, GPs were enlisted as local 'Panel doctors', and were paid an annual capitation fee per patient [39]. Despite its limitations, this important precursor to the NHS allowed patients to consider basic healthcare as a real possibility rather than an out-of-reach privilege.

With the establishment of more widespread primary care amongst low income workers, hospitals became more specialised and less about housing the ill and dying poor. In 1920, Lord Dawson's report into future healthcare provision built on this progress by providing an early blueprint for the NHS. Suggesting that hospitals became linked under a single administrative umbrella, the Dawson commission also foresaw the collation of community primary care and multidisciplinary services within health centres [40]. It was considered that GPs would offer general healthcare, with 'complex' cases referred for hospital management.

The next major advance came about in 1948, in the wake of destruction and privation wrought by World War II. The foundation of the National Health Service represented a huge shift overnight, offering the radical idea of socialised healthcare to the entire UK population which would be free of charge at the point of use. For the first time, any patient could be seen and treated without regard to their ability to pay.

'In this comprehensive scheme—quite the most ambitious adventure in the care of national health that any country has seen—it will inevitably be you, and the other professions with you, on whom everything depends. My job is to give you all the facilities, resources, apparatus, and help I can, and then to leave you alone as professional men and women to use your skill and judgment without hindrance. Let us try to develop that partnership from now on.' (Aneurin Bevan) [41].

At the formation of the NHS, differences between primary and secondary care became reified (made more concrete) into formal structures. With hospital practice considered of higher status, two thirds of new GPs at that time would have preferred a hospital career [42]. General practice required no postgraduate training after the first postgraduate year. Churchill's physician, Lord Moran, infamously testified to his perception of the inferiority of GPs in his evidence to the Commission on dentists' and doctors' pay:

> "The CHAIRMAN: It has been put to us by a good many people that the two branches of the profession, general practitioners and consultants, are not senior or junior to one another but that they are level. Do you agree with that?
>
> Lord MORAN: I say emphatically 'No.' Could anything be more absurd? I was dean of St. Mary's Hospital Medical School for 25 years, and all the people of outstanding merit, with few exceptions, aimed to get on the staff. It was a ladder off which they fell. How can you say that people who fall off the ladder are the same as those who do not? I am the son of a general practitioner. Is there no ladder? What are they doing then? Why do they try to get these places? I do not think you will find a single dean of any medical school who will give contrary evidence." (Lord Moran) [42]

The consultants Lord Moran considered to be at the 'top of the ladder' accepted a role as salaried doctors within the NHS, with the proviso that they were allowed time to pursue private work. GPs, on the other hand, chose to maintain their independent contractor status to preserve their autonomy, sitting outside the NHS while providing its services [43].

Within a month, 90% of the UK population had registered with a GP. Primary care also became a gateway to secondary care, with GPs the gatekeepers controlling referral. In the early NHS years, the quality of general practice varied greatly, with some practitioners under considerable stress. Facilities could be poor, with professional isolation common. Most GPs were either single-handed (worked alone) or had one partner. The longstanding promise of relocation to modern health centres was yet to materialise [39].

In 1950, a report in the *Lancet* by Australian GP Joseph Collings was a turning point for change. Collings came to the UK to learn from the much-admired NHS, but reported 'the overall state of general practice is bad and still deteriorating,' describing sometimes dirty conditions and rusty old instruments [44]. As a direct response to Collings and to support professional standards, the College of General Practitioners (RCGP) was convened in 1952. It was granted a Royal Charter in 1972. Once established, the RCGP became a focal point for training and professionalism [45].

Rather than being perceived as the province of doctors 'falling off' the secondary care ladder, general practice became established as a specialty in its own right. Membership and Fellowship of the RCGP were recognised by the GMC from 1967. Academic Departments of General Practice began to be established, developing an evidence base of primary care literature. In 1981, a vocational training scheme began under the RCGP's remit. New GPs now had to have a minimum of three years' postgraduate training, rather than entering general practice immediately post registration [45].

Current Social and Cultural Contexts

The state of contemporary UK general practice is described in this section, discussing the nature of work, the defining concepts of uncertainty and complexity, and primary care as the main site of clinical generalism. These are the contexts within which doctors learn, work and engage with other professionals. Social and cultural contexts are where identities are fledged and develop, through ordinary everyday activities.

At the time of writing in 2020, the small business model of general practice is still the most common set-up, preserving the independent contractor status agreed on in 1948. Small groups of doctors work in limited partnerships to deliver care to patient populations of highly variable size. Primary care networks and practice federations have been developed as the small business model has come under increasing pressure. There are also indications that new GPs are less interested in the business aspect of practice [46], meaning that in future a model where GPs agree to be salaried to the NHS (or to private providers) may become more likely. In the meantime, GPs mainly fall into three categories: partners, GPs salaried to practices, and independent sessional GPs who are self-employed and work across multiple settings.

Some GP practices work from rented health trust premises, while others own private accommodation. Funding is loosely based on a per capita mode for core General Medical Services (GMS), taking into account practice demographics in terms of patient age and sex, additional patient needs such as long standing illnesses, patient 'turnover', geographical variation in staff costs and rurality (the Carr-Hill formula). Additional income is available through the Quality and Outcomes Framework, a pay-for-performance scheme based on the achievement of evidence-based clinical targets, such as measuring annual blood pressure and lipid levels in patients with diabetes. Practices may also participate in enhanced services depending on local priorities. These include contraception, certain vaccinations and minor surgery [47].

Most GP surgeries are open during working hours, approximately 8.30 a.m. to 6 p.m., Monday to Friday, with some undertaking extended hours on evenings and at weekends. Out-of-hours work is no longer compulsory at practice level, with individual GPs instead being employed by choice by dedicated out-of-hours service providers in separate arrangements to their daytime jobs. The structure of in-hours work roughly consists of morning and afternoon surgeries along with phone calls, home visits and administration.

Prior to the 2020 coronavirus pandemic, general practice in the UK was under significant and increasing pressure [48]. This was multifactorial, as a result of increasing workloads moved from secondary care, increasing patient numbers and morbidity, and increased therapeutic potential for many conditions. Public health work, such as vaccination and screening programmes, are also central parts of general practice. Staff numbers, particularly in rural areas, dropped precipitously and vocational training programmes began to struggle to recruit [49, 50]. The COVID-19 pandemic has ushered in a paradigm shift which has not at the time of publication (2022) fully settled [51]. Amongst the radical changes to practice are a move to total telephone triage, with no booked appointments and all patients speaking to the GP before booking. This has had an immediate effect on the numbers of patients being seen in person. It is likely that many other structural changes will play out in the years following the pandemic.

Each of these contexts is essential to understand as a background to a career in general practice. Just as GP trainees need to have a functional understanding of hospital contexts in which they are training, they must learn about the situated norms of general practice in order to find their place in this world.

FIGURED WORLDS

A popular sociocultural model for describing identity development in medical education is Lave and Wenger' s Communities of Practice (CoP) model, whereby learners develop skills, and at the same time, move towards the centre of their community [52]. For hospital GP trainees, however, GP trainees are not just peripheral participants, but are *marginal* to whatever community of practice they are working in, making this a less useful model to conceptualise the hospital component of GP training.

A useful alternative is Holland's *figured worlds theory*, and Holland and Lave's extension of it, *social practice theory* [11, 53]. These share several assumptions with the better-known CoP theory: a commitment to seeing learning as a social activity, the use of actual or verbal tools as mediators of action, and the importance of language in building the structures of human existence. These can be used to understand how trainees construct their professional identities and how they manage their work within the various different cultural surroundings of the hospital.

In this way of thinking, learning goes well beyond classrooms and encompasses all the different types of knowledge and skills accrued through life and work experience. Learning is really just a continuous process of self-development, and identity is closely linked as it is synonymous with normal everyday practices. Figured worlds theory considers that these are influenced by the interplay between life experiences *(history in person)* and sociocultural contexts. It is also a *discourse* theory, meaning that it prioritises language as the most important way of human meaning making. Language can accomplish all sorts of social activity, not just reflecting but also constructing thought. In other words, learning how to talk in a particular way also means learning how to *think* in a particular way.

A *figured world* is an imaginative idea of a particular cultural context, and a *figured identity* is an imagined future self within that world. They are based on typical narratives and constructed through stories (narratives). Figured worlds and identities contribute to what it might seem possible to achieve. A classic example in medicine is of widening participation in medical school. If the world of medicine seems only for well-off, white, middle-class students, then a Black student from an area of deprivation will find it difficult to figure an identity for themselves as a doctor. Similarly, a lack of GP experience and role modelling during medical school will make it hard for graduates to see themselves becoming a GP.

Alongside figured identities, which represent a future sense of self, sit positional identities, which are about being given a particular status and place by others. If you grow up being positioned as taking over your father's business, then this may seem much more achievable than another career. If you are a GP trainee being positioned as a second-class doctor within a hospital training post, then you may well come to internalise that feeling as part of your identity. Figured identities are how we perceive the possibilities of our futures, while positional identities represent how society and culture define which possibilities are open to us at all. Both are by nature highly politicised, being heavily influenced by large-scale discourses of power.

ENDURING STRUGGLES

Holland and Lave broaden the ideas in figured worlds theory into *social practice theory*. This widens the frame to focus on how people, with their own personal identities and histories, engage with larger, shared cultural identities and histories [53].

Where two cultural ideologies clash over a long period of time, conflict (known as *enduring struggle*) becomes embedded into the identities of both the larger culture and the individuals engaged in action. One key example is the 'Black Lives Matter' movement, which has become locked in an enduring dyadic struggle with the alternative 'All Lives Matter.' The former seeks recognition of the impact of slavery and institutional racism on Black people, while the latter seeks to elide them [54]. Enduring struggles like this one are written so large that they are essential sites for exploring identities. Identities come out of everyday practice, and at sites of enduring struggle, everyday practice has a special name: *local contentious practice*. Examples are the demonstrations and counter-demonstrations of the two movements. Local contentious practice helps to construct a strong sense of identity within the ideological struggle.

Throughout the empirical narratives in Chaps. 2 and 3, the tension and power dynamics between primary and secondary care can be seen as an example of enduring struggle. The conflict is historically, socially and culturally constructed, and draws participants on both sides into local contentious practice. This phenomenon is explored more fully in Chap. 4.

INTRODUCING THE STORIES

In the following two chapters, narratives are presented from empirical research into developing GP identities. In the first chapter, seven junior doctors based in hospital as part of their GP training elicit important issues of conflict and identity. In the second chapter, an eighth doctor's story illustrates the evolution of her identity over the course of two years, as she moves from hospital-based into community-based GP training.

Narrative is used here as a privileged instance of language use between people. Through stories, people can connect past, present and future to make sense of life experiences [55]. Narratives, framed in this way, reconstitute as well as represent information. All the participants gave informed consent to participate in narrative interviews, and all were training within the Northern Ireland deanery between 2013–15. Seven identified as female and one as male. Analysis focuses on thematic content and linguistic processes within these stories (an approach known as *experience-centred narrative analysis* [56]). Narratives are situated in their multiple contexts, and the social work undertaken within them is acknowledged as these trainees try to understand their world and their own place in it.

REFERENCES

1. General Practice National Recruitment Office. The GP Training Programme. [Internet]. [cited 2020 Dec 22]. https://gprecruitment.hee.nhs.uk/Recruitment/Training.
2. Sabey A, Hardy H. Views of newly-qualified GPs about their training and preparedness: lessons for extended generalist training. Br J Gen Pract [Internet] 2015 Apr 1;65(633):e270. http://bjgp.org/content/65/633/e270.abstract.
3. Alberti H, Banner K, Collingwood H, Merritt K. 'Just a GP': a mixed method study of undermining of general practice as a career choice in the UK. BMJ Open [Internet] 2017 Nov [cited 2020 Jun 10];7(11):e018520. http://bmjopen.bmj.com/lookup/doi/10.1136/bmjopen-2017-018520.
4. Pereira Gray DJ. Just a GP. Gale Memorial Lecture. J R Coll Gen Pr. 1979;30(213):231–9.
5. Wass V, Gregory S. Not 'just' a GP: a call for action. Br J Gen Pract [Internet]. 2017 Apr [cited 2020 Jun 10];67(657):148–149. http://bjgp.org/lookup/doi/10.3399/bjgp17X689953.
6. Merrett A, Jones D, Sein K, Green T, Macleod U. Attitudes of newly qualified doctors towards a career in general practice: a qualitative focus group study. Br

J Gen Pract [Internet]. 2017 Apr 1;67(657):e253. http://bjgp.org/content/67/657/e253.abstract.

7. GPPS_2020_National_infographic_PUBLIC.pdf [Internet]. [cited 2020 Dec 22]. http://gp-patient.co.uk/downloads/2020/GPPS_2020_National_infographic_PUBLIC.pdf.

8. Brooks JV. Hostility during training: historical roots of primary care disparagement. Ann Fam Med [Internet]. 2016 Sep 1;14(5):446. http://www.annfammed.org/content/14/5/446.abstract.

9. Erikson EH. Identity and the life cycle. New York: W.W. Norton & Company; 1980.

10. Goffman E. The presentation of self in everyday life. London: Doubleday; 1959.

11. Holland DC. Identity and agency in cultural worlds. Cambridge, Mass: Harvard University Press; 1998.

12. Gee JP. Discourse, small d, big D. in: the international Encyclopedia of language and social interaction [internet]. Am Cancer Soc. 2015:1–5. https://onlinelibrary.wiley.com/doi/abs/10.1002/9781118611463.wbielsi016

13. Pownall H. Neoliberalism, austerity and the health and social care act 2012: the coalition Government's programme for the NHS and its implications for the public sector workforce. Ind Law J [Internet]. 2013 Dec 1 [cited 2020 Dec 22];42(4):422–433. https://doi.org/10.1093/indlaw/dwt016.

14. Fine B, Saad-Filho A. Thirteen things you need to know about neoliberalism. Crit Sociol [Internet]. 2016 Aug 19 [cited 2020 dec 22];43(4–5):685–706. https://doi.org/10.1177/0896920516655387.

15. Vernon J. The making of the neoliberal University in Britain. Crit Hist Stud [Internet]. 2018 Sep 1 [cited 2020 Dec 22];5(2):267–280. https://doi.org/10.1086/699686.

16. McArdle J. Medical training pathway [internet]. [cited 2020 Dec 22]. https://www.bma.org.uk/advice-and-support/studying-medicine/becoming-a-doctor/medical-training-pathway.

17. UK Foundation Programme. 2019 F2 Career Destinations Survey. UKFPO; 2020.

18. General Medical Council. Specialty destination [Internet]. Specialty destination. 2020 [cited 2020 Dec 22]. https://www.gmc-uk.org/education/reports-and-reviews/progression-reports/specialty-destination.

19. NHS England. General Practice Forward View [Internet]. NHS England; 2016 [cited 2020 Dec 22]. https://www.england.nhs.uk/wp-content/uploads/2016/04/gpfv.pdf.

20. Madan A, Manek N, Gregory S. General practice: the heart of the NHS. Br J Gen Pract [Internet]. 2017 Apr 1;67(657):150. http://bjgp.org/content/67/657/150.abstract.

21. Marchand C, Peckham S. Addressing the crisis of GP recruitment and retention: a systematic review. Br J Gen Pract J R Coll Gen Pract [Internet].

2017/03/13 ed. 2017 Apr;67(657):e227–e237. https://pubmed.ncbi.nlm.
nih.gov/28289014.
22. Verma P, Ford JA, Stuart A, Howe A, Everington S, Steel N. A systematic
review of strategies to recruit and retain primary care doctors. BMC Health
Serv Res [Internet] 2016 Apr 12;16:126–6. https://pubmed.ncbi.nlm.nih.
gov/27067255.
23. Alberti H, Randles HL, Harding A, McKinley RK. Exposure of undergradu-
ates to authentic GP teaching and subsequent entry to GP training: a quanti-
tative study of UK medical schools. Br J Gen Pract [Internet]. 2017 Apr
1;67(657):e248. http://bjgp.org/content/67/657/e248.abstract.
24. Vaidya HJ, Emery AW, Alexander EC, McDonnell AJ, Burford C, Bulsara
MK. Clinical specialty training in UK undergraduate medical schools: a retro-
spective observational study. BMJ Open [Internet]. 2019 Jul 1;9(7):e025403.
http://bmjopen.bmj.com/content/9/7/e025403.abstract.
25. Health Service Journal, Geometric Results Inc. Brexit and the NHS workforce: a guide for healthcare leaders [Internet]. HSJ; 2019. https://www.hsj.
co.uk/workforce/brexit-and-the-nhs-workforce-a-guide-for-healthcare-
leaders/7024658.article.
26. Kmietowicz Z. Doctors protest against "hostile environment" immigration
policy spreading to NHS. BMJ [Internet] 2018 May 2;361:k1953. http://
www.bmj.com/content/361/bmj.k1953.abstract.
27. World Health Organisation. Urgent health challenges for the next decade
[Internet]. 2020. https://www.who.int/news-room/photo-story/photo-
story-detail/urgent-health-challenges-for-the-next-decade.
28. Bliss M. William Osler: a life in medicine. Toronto: University of Toronto
Press; 1999.
29. Aira M, Mäntyselkä P, Vehviläinen A, Kumpusalo E. Occupational isolation
among general practitioners in Finland. Occup Med [Internet]. 2010 Sep 1
[cited 2020 Dec 22];60(6):430–435. https://doi.org/10.1093/occ-
med/kqq082.
30. Royal College of General Practitioners. First 5 [Internet]. 2020. rcgp.org.
uk/first5.
31. Giles S. Just family. Can Fam Physicoan. 53(7):1212.
32. Beaulieu M, Dory V, Pestiaux D, Pouchain D, Rioux M, Rocher G, et al.
What does it mean to be a family physician? Exploratory study with family
medicine residents from 3 countries. Can Fam Physicoan. 2009;55:e14–20.
33. O'Shea E. Extension of training for general practice: a review of the evidence.
Educ Prim Care. 2009;20(2):15–20.
34. Scallan S, Lyon-Maris J. The educational impact of COVID-19: views from
UK GP educators and trainees. Educ Prim Care [Internet]. 2020 Sep
2;31(5):328–329. https://doi.org/10.1080/14739879.2020.1806736.

35. Mol A, Berg M. Differences in medicine: Unravellingr practices, techniques and bodies. Durham: Duke University Press; 1998.
36. Bakhtin MM. The dialogic imagination: four essays. Austin: University of Texas Press; 1981.
37. The National archives. National Health Insurance [Internet]. 2020 [cited 2020 Dec 21]. https://www.nationalarchives.gov.uk/cabinetpapers/themes/national-health-insurance.htm.
38. REPORT OF THE Royal Commission on the poor Laws and Relief of distress. Br Med J [Internet]. 1909 Feb 27;1(2513):545. http://www.bmj.com/content/1/2513/545.abstract
39. Kmietowicz Z. A century of general practice. BMJ [Internet]. 2006 Jan 7;332(7532):39–40. https://pubmed.ncbi.nlm.nih.gov/16399738.
40. Future Provision Of Medical Services. Lord Dawson On The Consultative Council's Report. 1920;1(3102):800–2.
41. The new NHS: message to the medical profession from the minister of health. BMJ [Internet]. 1998 Jul 4;317(7150):72. http://www.bmj.com/content/317/7150/72.2.abstract.
42. Royal Commission on doctors' and dentists' remuneration. Lord Moran's evidence. Br Med J. 1958;1:27–30.
43. The King's Fund. Quality of care in general practice. Independent inquiry report, chapter two: the evolving role and nature of general practice in England [Internet]. The King's Fund; 2011. https://www.kingsfund.org.uk/sites/default/files/field/field_related_document/gp-inquiry-report-evolving-role-nature-2mar11.pdf.
44. The Collings Report. Orig Publ Vol 1 Issue 6604 [Internet]. 1950 Mar 25;255(6604):547–9. http://www.sciencedirect.com/science/article/pii/S0140673650904624.
45. Royal College of General Practitioners. History of the College [Internet]. 2012. https://www.rcgp.org.uk/about-us/the-college/who-we-are/history-heritage-and-archive/history-of-the-college.aspx.
46. Iacobucci G. New business models would boost GP partnerships, says review. BMJ [Internet]. 2019 Jan 15;364:l222. http://www.bmj.com/content/364/bmj.l222.abstract.
47. Moberly T, Stahl-Timmins W. QOF now accounts for less than 10% of GP practice income. BMJ [Internet]. 2019 Apr 2;365:l1489. http://www.bmj.com/content/365/bmj.l1489.abstract.
48. Fisher RF, Croxson CH, Ashdown HF, Hobbs FR. GP views on strategies to cope with increasing workload: a qualitative interview study. Br J Gen Pract [Internet]. 2017 Feb 1;67(655):e148. http://bjgp.org/content/67/655/e148.abstract.

49. Taylor M. Why is there a shortage of doctors in the UK? Bull R Coll Surg Engl [Internet]. 2020 Mar 1 [cited 2020 Dec 22];102(3):78–81. https://doi.org/10.1308/rcsbull.2020.78.

50. Lawson E, Kumar S. The Wass report: moving forward 3 years on. Br J Gen Pract [Internet]. 2020 Apr 1;70(693):164. http://bjgp.org/content/70/693/164.abstract.

51. Johnston JL, Hart N. Primary care education in the time of COVID: embodiment, identity and loss. Educ Prim Care [Internet]. 2020 Oct 28:1–4. https://doi.org/10.1080/14739879.2020.1837020

52. Lave J, Wenger E. Situated learning: legitimate peripheral participation. Cambridge: Cambridge University Press; 1991.

53. Holland D, Lave J. History in person: enduring struggles, contentious practice, intimate identities. Santa Fe: School of American Research Press; 2001.

54. Carney N. All lives matter, but so does race: black lives matter and the evolving role of social media. Humanity Soc [Internet]. 2016 Apr 13 [cited 2020 Dec 22];40(2):180–199. https://doi.org/10.1177/0160597616643868.

55. Ricoeur P. Time and narrative volume 1. Chicago: University of Chicago Press; 1990.

56. Squire C. Experience-centred and culturally-oriented approaches to narrative. In: Andrews M, Squire C, Tamboukou M, editors. Doing narrative research. London: Sage; 2008.

CHAPTER 2

GP Identities in Hospital

Abstract This chapter outlines narrative accounts of lived experience, acquired during empirical interviews with a small group of GP trainees working in NHS hospitals. The tensions embedded in their daily work can be seen both to impact their learning about themselves and to manifest historical dynamics in a way which maintains conflict. Those who offered their experiences can be seen to engage in complex identity work within layers of social context and cultural 'rules.'

Keywords GP • Identity • Postgraduate training • Medical education • Narrative analysis • NHS

This is the first of two chapters showcasing the narratives of GP trainees working in hospital, and explores how they are confronted with the tensions between primary and secondary care within their everyday work. Trainees are faced with a decision as to whether to accept or contest the idea of primary care as of lower status. Based in hospital communities of practice, trainees contribute to these as is expected of them, but also construct their own, alternative community around being future GPs. In the overwhelming female narratives (only one participant is male), the gendering of specialty choice also becomes clear. All the trainees used these interviews, which were minimally structured and conducted by two experienced GPs, as a way of making sense of their experiences and practising their GP identities. Multiple different voices can be read in their narratives, representing their own present view of themselves, their past and future selves and others who they encounter through the course of their work. Pseudonyms are used throughout. All the participants in this chapter were white. Seven originated from Northern Ireland, and the eighth, Maria, whose story appears in the following chapter, was from Co Donegal in the Republic of Ireland.

Deciding to Become a GP

Three trainees had had F2 GP placements (Kerry, Clare and Emma). They joined GP training directly from the foundation programme, together with one other trainee, Laura. The other three trainees (Niamh, Louise and David) had trained in hospital specialties first. At the time of interview, they were only a few months into their GP training scheme and all were working in hospital posts (ranging across Emergency Medicine, Cardiology, Psychiatry and Obstetrics and Gynaecology).

Kerry had originally chosen to study medicine with the intention of eventually becoming a GP. Her identity as a medical student and doctor is already tied in with primary care, which fits her understanding of other aspects of herself:

> 'When I was at school and sort of making decisions about what to do GP was the sort of thing that I'd always thought about and whilst I was interested in medicine I knew I was going to university to study, it was always an end point that I thought I would be more suited to a GP, I just felt with my own personality.' (Kerry)

For the others, the decision came later. The F2 GP placement was pivotal for the trainees who had undertaken it. They were able to develop mentoring relationships with other doctors in primary care and develop their sense of how primary care works. More senior GPs were often seen as role models and were influential, as Emma describes here in talking about discussing her career choice with the GP partners:

> 'The partners were getting very stressed and the older partners were just like, this [GP] is awful, this is horrendous, don't do this ... and my trainer was like, I love it, do do it, do do it and she was lovely and I just kind of—I think I was very similar to her in a way you know.' (Emma)

Emma sees something in her trainer which she would like to achieve for herself. She uses direct reported speech (quoting the voices of the partners and her trainer as if they were speaking) which creates a vivid sense of the characters, with the positive viewpoint ultimately winning.

Role models were also important for David and Louise, but through family and friends rather than professional experience. Both of them tried other training schemes before entering GP training, but neither of them had worked in primary care before. Interestingly, both of them had influential personal relationships with GPs (family doctors) in North America. They both saw the job as being more or less the same no matter where it was practised.

> 'I have an uncle in Canada who is a GP and is the best advertisement for his job and just loves, loves, loves his job. And goes in too early and does night time clinics and people only come to see him, they won't see any of the other GPs. … He was very bewildered at the idea of me doing psych [psychiatry] or anaesthetics, so I went in and did about three or four days with him and just saw patients and then he came behind me afterwards [to finish the consultation] and I was kind of converted.' (Louise)

Louise's narrative shows she thinks of her uncle as a role model. There is notable privilege in being able to access this type of family role model, and her experience would not be open to all postgraduates. Her work experience took place in Canada, so benefits from being somewhat exotic and outside the regular daily routines. It is worth mentioning the relationship that Northern Ireland and the Republic of Ireland have with North America, following the large waves of emigration there in the nineteenth and twentieth centuries [1]. This aspect is in the background of her narrative but might not be obvious to readers from other contexts.

Louise also follows the traditional discourse that doctors must have a commitment to medicine overriding other aspects of life. She is proud that her uncle is a popular GP, prioritising relational care, and works above and beyond, disregarding any home commitments he might have. Meanwhile the uncle is presented as a strong character, who sees GP as the only 'real' medical career and who helps her to safely try on a GP identity with the benefit of his good relationships with his patients. Her 'conversion' uses a religious metaphor as a way to emphasis its significance for her, and perhaps, like her uncle, seeing an importance to the work which almost borders on spiritual [2].

David also locates GP identity in patient relationships and is disparaging about hospital care:

'I have got a very good friend in Minnesota who's a GP, and I spent a lot of time back and forward with him and I loved that and he said, look it's great because there is a bit more getting to know people and you are not just doing something for them and dispatching them and forgetting about them.' (David)

This narrative references David's disillusion with medical efficiency discourse, which recasts patients' illness experiences within industrial terms [3]. The status of GPs in their communities is also important for him here. In the following narrative, he positions himself as fairly passive in his decision-making, which is influenced by others' hopes and expectations of him:

'And then it was even things like—family, neighbours, people started to come to me, and everything they came to me with were GP type things … and I thought I could see that they found the help valuable and then they started saying to me, oh you should be a GP.' (David)

Similar to Louise, David uses a metaphor which is semi-religious, depicting himself as having an innate skill which draws others to him, like a historical picture of a healer with acolytes sitting around him. As with Louise, medicine is approached with an almost spiritual awe which goes beyond a socially useful vocation. His paints his choice to be a GP as almost inevitable with little sense of personal agency.

For Niamh, who had spent time training in surgery, her decision to become a GP was met with negative reactions from friends and family:

'People think it's—have a perception that you are just sitting in an office all day … I don't think it's as mundane as maybe other people perceive it to be. And even family members who aren't medical would say, you know sure it's just a job where you see coughs and colds … there is a lot more depth to it than people realise you know.' (Niamh)

Although GPs are well-regarded by their patients, perhaps this narrative reflects additional status Niamh's family may have afforded to a surgical career. Surgeons are often considered to sit high up in the informal hierarchy of medical specialties [4]. Niamh, like David and Louise, had no previous experience of working in GP, but contests negative stereotypes.

Clare joined GP training straight after the foundation programme, and had completed an F2 placement in general practice. Part of her decision was influenced by what she saw as greater autonomy available to GPs. Like David, she is critical of hospital processes, recognising the influence of efficiency discourse and finding it restrictive in terms of patient-centred care delivery:

> 'There is a lot of pressure from bed managers and different things in hospitals that you just sometimes think that the patient's best interests aren't being put to the forefront. Whereas I don't know in GP you can kind of control that a little bit more.' (Clare)

The commitment in general practice to engaging in longitudinal relationships with patients is one of the most attractive aspects of the job for her. Clare prioritises relationships with patients, aligning herself with the values of primary care:

> 'I like the communication part of things, I like talking to people and that was the bit that I really enjoyed more than the other aspects of medicine … and I think you kind of get to know that over your foundation year, that those are the bits you like whenever you get to know someone, or if you have an unusual or interesting conversation with someone, or there is something difficult to kind of explain those are the bits I liked … that's where I fitted in and I didn't necessarily as much fit into the personality type that some doctors in hospitals have as much.' (Clare)

Clare's experience of the foundation scheme was formative in helping her make career choices. Clare mirrors Kerry in distinguishing between 'personalities' suited to hospital and community careers. The subtext of her comments on communication refers to the different ideologies and discursive practices of primary and secondary care, which she is already aware of. She is confident that she fits within the wider world of medicine but expresses her fundamental sense of not belonging in hospital.

All these trainees notably contrasted general practice careers to hospital practice. Primary care became a kind of foil which they used to contest hospital norms, imaginatively developing a narrativised, figured idea of their future medical careers beyond secondary care.

First Steps to a New Identity

The trainees had all been successful in a complex and rigorous admission process. Although the GP training scheme in Northern Ireland has variable numbers of applicants from year to year, following the trend in other parts of the UK, at the time these trainees had applied, GP training was oversubscribed and highly competitive. This meant that getting accepted was something to be proud of and a marker of status and identity. Even though they continued to work in hospitals after joining the scheme, there was an immediate shift in identity, as they were now GP trainees rather than simply junior hospital doctors.

Clare felt that the application process reflected the core pragmatism of general practice, and contrasted it against commerciality in selection for hospital general medicine training:

> 'I don't like doing things for the sake of it, you know a lot of other specialties there is a lot of tick box exercises and you have to do x amount of audits and people don't want to do these audits and they just do them for the sake of … the medicine interview where they are sort of picking at your CV. … I don't mind doing things that I enjoy to progress, but people go off and do all these courses and spend all this money and they are not interested in doing it.' (Clare)

Clare constructs success in secondary care training applications as a type of status which can be bought with time and money, rather than reflecting a true vocation. She manages to position herself outside a competitive race in which tick-box achievements seem to have more value than a commitment to patients. Already she has a strong GP identity which is presented as a counter-culture to that of junior doctors in hospitals.

Louise began the application process while she was working in a non-training hospital post in Australia. This remains a popular choice for junior doctors straight after the F2 year. Louise is surprised by the sense of community around the GP application process:

> 'I couldn't really afford the money to come home twice in six weeks to do the MCQ and then do the interview, so … I went to the, it was like a driving test place in Hyde Park [in Sydney] and went to the interview and met all these people from Northern Ireland that I didn't even know were there. … They were all applying for GP somewhere in the UK so that was quite funny. And yeah then came home for the interview and was surprised to see lots of

faces of people who had been my seniors in different specialties, I was sitting beside a surgical reg and there was a girl who had been an anaesthetic reg on my left and it kind of made me feel like I wasn't sitting there with a bunch of F2s who were fresh faced and, or bushy tailed bright eyed.'(Louise)

At this stage, Louise is more ambivalent than Clare about her possible identity as a GP, and she is not as negative as Clare about hospital practice. The fact that more senior hospital doctors are also applying for GP training seems to give her decision legitimacy. She also connects again with the long history of Irish emigration, finding a sense of community in shared experience of being away from home. For context, Northern Ireland is unusual in having a choice of cultural identities: British, Irish, Northern Irish or a combination of any of these [5]. The longstanding emigration narrative becomes quickly entwined with her new professional identity. In fact, spending time out of postgraduate training in Australia has become so popular for doctors from the island of Ireland that Bennett characterises it as a paradigmatic trajectory (a typical developmental path within a community of practice) [6].

Once trainees had completed the selection processes, there followed a time of uncertainty and contingency planning while they waited to hear if they had been successful. This was a challenging time when they were forced to consider alternative possible future selves. Junior doctors who are not part of training schemes are anecdotally considered lower status, meaning that it was better to accept an offer they weren't sure about than to end up with nothing. GP training was Kerry's first choice, but she also applied to psychiatry as a back-up plan. When she receives acceptance to both, she is confronted with a dilemma:

'I got my psych offer I think the day before my GP interview, so at that point I was quite happy going into GP knowing well, if the interview doesn't go well I would still take the psych job, but ended up very fortunately getting an offer for both and it was a stressful enough twelve hours making a decision, but I think in my heart of hearts GP was the way forward and certainly have no regrets now … the offer came through for GP that I realised I can't turn this down, you know this opportunity might not come up again.' (Kerry)

Here, Kerry is reflecting, in an understated way, on how her entire career might hang on this one decision. The subtext here is that training offers in the Northern Ireland (NI) context are usually only given once, making it hard for her to change her mind. She thinks very carefully about what it might look like to be a psychiatrist and what it might look like to be a GP, and in the end feels that general practice is closer to her core sense of self.

In contrast, GP training was the back-up plan for Laura. She accepted her place only after not being accepted to hospital medicine training. In this narrative, she struggles a little with the new GP identity:

'I don't know, I applied for [acute hospital] medicine and GP, initially wanting to go for medicine and then didn't get a core medical job right away, and at the time whenever the jobs came out, I was working in the Accident and Emergency department (A&E), and I'd met a lot of GPs there and you know the GPs who have a special interest in A&E and I talked to them and they really turned me on to the idea. So I whenever I got the GP job I took it em, and ... yeah, I don't know.' (Laura)

Accepting a place in GP training was a pragmatic choice which allows her to safeguard her social position. Laura had no F2 experience in primary care and had not been planning a GP career, but was influenced by colleagues who were experienced GPs working in A&E. This is a special interest for some qualified GPs and for Laura, who valued hospital work, may have increased the legitimacy of GP careers. However, she still expresses some uncertainty about the choice, and this comes up again in later parts of her narrative. In contrast, Niamh, who had been a surgical trainee, is proud of her success which has increased her sense of confidence in her choice:

'Even some of the F2s might come and ask you what it is like to be a GP trainee or what the GP application was like, you know because they might be considering it now ... you do feel a sense of nearly accomplishment because the F2s are preparing to apply at this time, they know or they have maybe heard from other people how rigorous an application it is and then they maybe come and ask for advice on how you find the process and how you got through the process and things like that.' (Niamh)

All of a sudden, Niamh is a role model herself as a result of her new 'insider' status. There is a sharp contrast here with the negative attitudes that she spoke about earlier from family and friends. This positive feedback on her new professional self helps her to consolidate her commitment to general practice.

These narratives show that tentative GP identities start with thinking about the application process, long before actually starting on the job. In order to apply, the trainees had to figure themselves imaginatively within the GP world. Each trainee brings their own personal experiences and ideas with them (their *history in person* [7]) as they start out on this professional journey.

RECONCILING PAST AND PRESENT SELVES

Two elements of previous work experience were relevant for trainees. All three (Clare, Emma and Kerry) who had done F2 placements were noticeably confident in their career choice. This might well reflect their F2 experience, or perhaps that they were interested in GP at the time of applying for F2 schemes. For the three who had experience in hospital training (David, Louise and Niamh), their decisions and identities were not so clear cut.

Louise had first applied to anaesthetic training but had not been offered a place. She then chose to work in psychiatry training (her contingency plan) as she had enjoyed it in F2, but found she was positioned differently as a specialty trainee:

'I started psych [psychiatry] training, knew within five or six months that I missed [acute] medicine and clinical examination. And didn't feel like I was allowed to use any of the medicine that I had learned, which was quite frustrating because there was loads of medicine as well, because there's so many comorbidities. And I couldn't do anything, I kept having to send them out [refer to other hospital doctors], so I knew pretty sharpish that I wasn't going to do that.' (Louise)

Louise reflects here on the culture of psychiatry, which she experienced as separate from other parts of medicine. The extent of this was such that as a psychiatry trainee (rather than an F2 just visiting), she would have to choose between identities as a psychiatrist or physician, but not hold both together. Despite perceiving that she had the appropriate skills, she was expected to refer, rather than treat, physical conditions. Resultantly, she left psychiatry training and took a break working in Australia. Below, she frames her decision not to apply to GP earlier as a result of not having had an F2 placement. Discursively, Louise is defensive against any perception that she has not been totally committed to GP:

'Just whatever way my application worked out I didn't get that rotation, so ... But I know for a fact that probably 80 per cent of the people who did GP as an F2 went onto to either do it straight away or took a year out and then have come back and done it. ... So, I am fairly sure if I had done it as an F2 I would have gone into it straight away.' (Louise)

Niamh, like Louise, was influenced by a positive F2 experience and was accepted to surgical training straight from the foundation programme. Once working in surgery, she became concerned that it was incompatible with her plans for a family:

'Coming out of F2 I applied for surgery, but I think maybe I wasn't thinking you know ten, twenty, thirty years down the line, I think I liked it at the time and just applied for it at the time. So that is how I ended up in surgical training, because I suppose now it seems strange because surgery is such a different specialty to general practice, but I didn't really know what I wanted to do. ... I suppose in my mind I was thinking of a job for the next year and the next year and the next year but I suppose I hadn't broadened my thoughts to what would suit me, what might have been appropriate at 24 years of age might not have suited me at 40 or 50.' (Niamh)

Like Louise, Niamh is defending her choice here to try something else and then enter GP training. She had left surgical training after being influenced by gendered career expectations in surgical training, and the opposite gendered expectations (that GP is a flexible job for a woman) influence her decision to become a GP. Niamh acknowledges the gendered nature of both these specialties:

'I suppose just like you wouldn't want to admit it always, but as a female you do have to consider things and that was my perspective anyway that maybe at 25 years of age [working shifts] don't affect your life really, but I didn't want to do another ten or fifteen years of shift work which is demanding on your time and your kind of emotional availability and everything else, and so—and me personally I want to have a family down the line and I didn't think it was going to be compatible to that, you know as much as I would want it to be.' (Niamh)

This narrative shows Niamh thinking deeply about how her professional self might mesh with her other identities in future. She enjoys surgery but sees herself as needing to make space for future family life—a decision based on the historical structures of surgery which, arguably, her male surgical colleagues will not have had to make. Her use of language is carefully chosen to neutralise any perceived emotion or stereotypical femininity, reinforcing the idea she presents that these traits are unwelcome in surgery or indeed in medicine.

In surgery, there is a long tradition of women passing as 'one of the boys' [8]. Like Louise, Niamh finds that a specialty she enjoyed as an F2 passing through has different connotations as a committed trainee. She worked hard to fit in in the culture of surgical training and embraced her place in their community of practice.

'I think in any surgical job you just have to throw yourself into the job because the time is so demanding … the colleagues that you are working with you know are of a certain personality type so you kind of, you just have to throw yourself into it but if you do, and I did, you do get a lot from it. … I mean you were very busy all the time, kind of a lot was demanded from you, you know, but I think you know it makes you become more resilient and it makes you become more—better at kind of acting on your feet and making decisions and becoming a more independent clinician whether that is in surgery or in any other specialty. You know, so it's character building in a way.' (Niamh)

The learning that Niamh took away from surgery reflects a classic individualist narrative of medicine, where it is important to stand on one's own feet, and difficult experiences need to be briskly dismissed. Later, she speaks about using her technical skills in minor surgery, so her GP career will let her maintain aspects of her surgeon identity. This contrasts with Louise's characterisation of psychiatry as limited. Niamh undertook a year working in acute medicine after leaving surgical training, and feels that she is entering GP with a more mature attitude:

'I kind of felt that maybe in retrospect if I had done that kind of rigorous interview process just coming out of F2 I might not have done as well, because I think a lot of the skills I was able to demonstrate in the interview process I had actually learned in the two years post-foundation training and I think that is why I was able to come across in a certain way. And I maybe had gained a certain level of insight and maturity that I didn't have in F2, so I think it actually helped me in the long run you know.' (Niamh)

David, in contrast to Niamh and Louise, spent two years out of clinical work as a Health Board manager. This would have been a very unusual choice at his career stage. He was keen to re-enter clinical training but disliked hospital medicine. David sees GP careers as having more room for personal agency:

> 'So that [his Health Board job] was done as out of programme for a year, then they asked me to stay on for another year and I did, and then after two years, during that time I decided I didn't want to go back. And I'd had a chat with various people in the deanery about that ... she said let me suggest why you don't want to do it, it's because of lack of autonomy. You would rather be a GP because it's a faster route to being an autonomous practitioner.' (David)

Just as when talking about making the decision to apply, David presents himself as having been influenced and encouraged by others. Despite this professed lack of agency, he places a high value on professional autonomy, which seems to him more accessible through general practice. Historically, GPs, as self-employed small business owners, have been seen to be more autonomous than consultants directly salaried to the NHS. David's language is intensely negative in referring to hospital training:

> 'We had a reunion and all my friends who had went into GP were the happiest of the bunch. People who did medicine weren't happy, the surgical people weren't—the people generally who were in hospital were not happy. ... I think it is probably that sort of disempowerment and lack of autonomy, so you go in and you work in a big machine and you're a small cog, you are treated like the dogsbody sometimes, you are just there to churn out activity and get work done. Your—the training is atrocious, I mean the training that I got in medicine was atrocious. Anything I learned, I learned myself.' (David)

Here David is constructing himself as contesting a repressive system based on efficiency and conformity. For the first time, he gives a strong sense of personal agency, drawing a picture of a struggle of an individual against the system. For all three of the trainees who had tried hospital training before coming to GP, there was a process of self-discovery through disillusionment. They all see GP work as allowing them to keep something of their old interests and identity. General practice is the option which will get them out of hospital, and it is constructed in opposition to hospital rather than on its own terms.

None of these three have experience of working as GPs, so they have had to make high-stakes career decisions without being fully informed about what working in primary care really looks like. They are all making a paradigm shift from secondary to primary care, and this is not without risk.

OUTSIDER IDENTITIES IN HOSPITAL

One key difference between speciality and GP trainees is that GP training means starting from scratch with each rotation, since very different skills might be needed between, for example, psychiatry and emergency medicine. Specialty trainees still move contexts and teams, but they can build on and consolidate their skills. GP trainees are always by definition at the margins of the community of practice. They are cultural visitors, which can be uncomfortable: unlike F2s, they can find themselves positioned as lower status by their peers and supervisors. Tensions can arise between service commitment and training needs which may not be fully recognised by hospital staff.

Niamh found her consultant supervisors were supportive of core training days which needed study leave, but felt that this was not often the situation:

'Our consultants in A&E are very much like, when are your GP training days, and even if our rota goes short and they have to get in a locum to cover they will move mountains you know to get us to go out to them, because they recognise the importance of them. Whereas in another specialty in the same hospital you know it was almost like you can either take it as annual leave or you can't go, or only if it suits the rota or the service provision, so it wasn't anywhere near the same emphasis that they were a GP trainee and therefore should go out to their GP training days, it was just that they were an SHO [senior house officer] on their service and they just had to deal with it as such.' (Niamh)

The fact that study leave was not always possible for essential training, despite dates being published months in advance, emphasises the in-between and ephemeral status of GP trainees in hospital. Their early professional identity had to sometimes come second to their service provision role. They are adaptable because they had to be and work hard to be accepted:

> 'I think the GP trainees kind of adapt to whatever they are doing and just muck in and get on with things as well as everyone else.' (Clare)

Even while continuing to contribute to hospital teams, trainees held on tight to their fledgling GP identities. Clare reflects here on the transitory nature of her hospital post and, in contrast, the fundamental nature of her GP identity:

> 'I don't feel like I am a psychiatrist, sometimes I feel like I am pretending to be a psychiatrist. … I think you have to remind yourself you are a GP trainee and there is some things in psychiatry that it's useful to be a GP trainee for, especially the medical things. … I kind of went in with the perspective of, right I am going to look at this like they were coming to see me in the GP practice I was working in last year and what would I do if I saw them there. … I kind of thought I will just look at it that way as if I am their GP nearly because they can't really go out to see their GP.' (Clare)

The idea Clare expresses so elegantly is that in passing so well as a hospital doctor, her fundamental GP identity could be lost. She draws on F2 experience to frame herself as a GP in psychiatry rather than a psychiatrist. This internal dialogue is used as a way to create space to practise her identity, in a very patient-centred way. This is noticeably different from Louise, who felt powerless to treat patients more globally as a psychiatry trainee. Although the post is the same, the different positions are afforded different possibilities within the specialty culture.

Similarly, Kerry draws on the GP identity she developed in her F2 placement to help her through challenging times working in areas she has little affinity for:

> 'I think knowing in the end that you are a generalist and not a specialist of anything that you see or come across now … you just have to keep that mindset in the days of A&E when it's, yeah you're feeling a bit down with it all.' (Kerry)

Kerry is showing a clear commitment to clinical generalism and GP work. The hospital part of training is a means to an end. There is a suggestion that Kerry does not feel any sense of belonging in this post. In one sense, though, the difficulties she experiences help to mediate her identity as a GP. She draws on this identity to advocate for her own training needs:

> '[Senior staff] don't really know what stage we're all at sometimes, because they don't know that I'm GP training and the rest are A&E training. I try and tell them all, so we kind of know at the time … I do try and make that distinction because I think it's probably more fair … I have to say that yes, I'm a GP trainee but at the moment I'm in A&E and I just have to give myself to it, and give my all and learn from it, and I'm sort of looking at it with a GP perspective.' (Kerry)

The hospital component of GP training can be seen here to be different from hospital specialty training, and yet also different from GP practice-based training. Often, trainees are forging a difficult path without clinical supervisors having a clear idea of their educational needs. They are on the edge of communities of practice by necessity, while their hospital peers make inroads into the centre. They have to find safe spaces to develop their identities, because these are not automatically provided.

ALTERNATIVE COMMUNITIES

In this uncomfortable environment, trainees connected with each other to form an alternative GP training community. Even though they were dispersed across different hospital departments, they had a shared goal and shared activity. The alternative community centred around core GP training days, when they had half or full day release from their service jobs to learn about aspects of general practice. Although these days usually took place within the hospital, they were always facilitated by an experienced GP and were an important forum for identity work through conversation.

> 'They remind you that you are a GP trainee and that you are not a psychiatry trainee and I really enjoy them and think they are very beneficial actually … it does, it reminds you what you are doing, it feels nice, more so than F1 and F2 that you are in a training programme and that you actually feel involved.' (Clare)

Niamh describes how this community became a safe space in which to swap 'war stories,' a way to make sense of difficult experiences and to consolidate GP identities. These sessions were essential breathing spaces which refortified trainees to go back to their normal jobs.

> 'It's quite a good little support network ... the GP core group tend—we tend to kind of stick together ... we kind of support each other because we know that it's not the ideal specialty for us, but we can see why it's obviously beneficial for GP trainees to work there. ... We kind of did, you know we made kind of rules of the group at the very start to say that you know it is a place where you could come to, to vent or to you know tell others who are in the same boat you know things that have happened ... there are some funny stories.' (Niamh)

Friends who chose to be interviewed together, Emma and Laura discuss a war story here which illustrates the gap they perceive between everyday life in hospital posts and their end goal of becoming GPs:

> 'L: I lysed a STEMI [ST elevation myocardial infarction] was undecided but the patient was allergic to aspirin so I didn't give them aspirin and then they reinfarcted [had a further heart attack] and then I felt really bad, they needed to be bluelighted [sent to the tertiary centre by emergency ambulance], and I reflected on that, and then I was like, what am I reflecting on that for, it's not related to GP in any way whatsoever, it's a STEMI...
> E: What do you take from that, how do you put the GP spin on it?' (Laura, Emma)

Laura is clearly describing a sense of distress here. She uses the social language of secondary care jargon to tell her story: in lay language, she treated someone with a heart attack but it was unsuccessful, resulting in a second heart attack and an emergency admission to a tertiary centre for stent insertion. She is worried that her decision to withhold aspirin due to a stated allergy was wrong.

Despite reflecting on the incident, she can't make sense of it, and it has caused a secondary conflict as she cannot find a way to relate it to her GP training. Her use of jargon is a claim to belonging in the hospital community she is working in. Without discussing with a mentor, her distress over this incident may well remain unresolved. Emma, who has a more settled sense of herself as a GP, also worries over how hospital experiences can be made relevant to her longer-term goals. In the attempt to relate hospital experiences to general practice, Laura and Emma are referencing the mandatory reflection element of their e-portfolio, in which trainees are meant to record their progress during each attachment. This is supervised by a GP trainer outside the hospital, and so gives trainees a rare space for dialogue with general practice.

'You kind of feel like somebody is taking in and trusting your training and even from the point of the portfolio my trainer is on it every week, putting comments on and stuff like that and you kind of feel like somebody is actually interested in what you are doing and how you are progressing.' (Clare)

Much of the journey of these trainees does not fit a traditional communities of practice model, where increasing competence moves learners towards the centre of the community. They have to find space to develop their identities (a *space of authoring* [9]) *between* different hospital communities.

Here, Emma refers to trainees who are more senior to her within the alternative community of hospital-based GP trainees. These doctors are now GP registrars (ST3s in the final year of training), who have left hospital to move into community practices. Their trajectory gives her a way of figuring her own future self:

'I think there's a real sense of like, community or something in GP training and it's going to those half days and you know everybody and it's really nice ... our half day, the ST3s are there at the same time, when they come in and I knew a few of them from rotations and it was just nice to see them and how they all got on and then they're coming back every week now in [hospital name], so you see them every day and I thought, that will be me in two years, you know, coming here on a Thursday and having my own GP day— it's nice.' (Emma)

Once trainees have finished the hospital component and are based in the community, their learning can follow a more recognisable trajectory. During their time in hospital, their identities within hospital specialties are temporary and necessary, but they retain a sense of themselves as belonging to the world of general practice. Ironically, it is their shared sense of not belonging which pulls them together.

What Makes a 'Good GP'?

Given that identities are developed socially and culturally, they are inevitably political. Identities determine the range of actions that people are enabled to take within their own cultural spaces, and so they help determine the power relationships that develop between individuals or groups. In turn, then, they influence whether existing structures of power are maintained or contested.

In Chap. 1, the historical inequality between primary and secondary care was explored. Although these GP trainees worked hard to develop spaces for their own agency within complex structural constraints, they were still subject to potential stigma and misunderstanding arising from persistent inequality:

> 'I find it hard that people are like, oh you sit on your bum all day and don't do very much and I think I find that a bit challenging ... sometimes the hospital doctors and people working in hospitals have that sort of perception.' (Clare)

GPs are, by definition, a minority in hospitals. Outside training, only a minority are likely to work in secondary care clinics (as GPs with a special interest (GPwSI)). Trainees' mentors and role models during secondary care placements must therefore be drawn mainly from hospital doctors, rather than GPs. Yet these mentors may never have worked in primary care, and may hold views which would be contested within primary care itself. Laura comments succinctly on this phenomenon:

> 'I get the impression people think you're a bit soft.' (Laura)

This is a piece of *intertextuality*—when one understanding is shaped by another. Here, the discourse referred to is the false logic that a focus is on relational care must mean that 'hard' (scientifically rigorous) medicine is not done.

Particularly problematic are trainees' experiences where hospital standards of good practice were applied directly from primary to secondary care without translation or attention to context. Clinical decision making is a key area of such conflict: secondary care decisions are mediated by performing tests, but this is only true to a limited extent in primary care. Emma, who has worked on both sides, expresses her frustration here with this fundamental misunderstanding:

'They don't understand what it's like to be sitting there and not have the bloods and not have the ECG and not have the x-ray and of course they can say the troponin's [cardiac blood test] negative, it's not, I'm like, the GP can't say that and I don't think people understand that. I don't think people understand that. I don't think there's enough understanding of that in hospital. I think they're very harsh on GPs.' (Emma)

Emma uses rhythm and repetition to underline her point, which is that GPs are vilified for sending patients to A&E. Yet she recognises what her hospital colleagues may not, which is that GP consultations are cross-sectional and limited in their use of tests. This is not feasibly achievable in primary care, where a diagnostic decision has to be made quickly on history, examination and basic testing. A patient with a negative troponin who can be sent home is easily seen as a waste of hospital time and resources in retrospect, yet the test is fundamental in making that decision.

Laura finds this kind of stigma particularly stinging, perhaps because she still feels something of the identity of a hospital doctor:

'Oh you're just a GP—I'm like, well no actually. Do you know if you want me to stick a needle in that knee I will, you know this isn't just something just for the medical trainees. Just cause I want to be a GP. All the regs and stuff are like, you're just a GP. It's like, not just!' (Laura)

As she did in her earlier narrative, Laura appropriates hospital language, and she focuses on the procedure, rather than the patient, to express her sense of belonging in hospital and to assert herself as an equal to the specialty trainees. Undertaking procedures is something she sees as a mediator of hospital identity and so this is a claim to status. The disembodied knee is a classic example of Foucault's clinical gaze and runs counter to the relational discourse of GP, which she felt caused her to be perceived as 'soft'.

In Louise's narrative, the stigma Laura and Emma have experienced directly is not quite so obvious:

'[A&E consultants] have kind of said all the GP trainees they are going to like take turns, but pop you into minors [minor injuries] and you just see for days on end, if you annoy me or piss me off I am going to put you in minors for a week and all you'll see is children and he was like after a week in there youse [you all] will all be amazing GPs, he was kind of like the more we give you the better, the less referrals we are going to get.' (Louise)

This is a more insidious way of expressing the same power dynamic. The consultants Louise speaks of are apparently trying to be helpful and humorous. This kind of hegemonic assumption is, however, very undermining. General practice is subtly demeaned as analogous to emergency department 'minors', and this in itself is depicted as somewhere A&E doctors dislike working. Even worse, the consultant feels he can define what a good GP is, and his sole criteria is not referring patients to hospital. Louise seems to accept this. Because the consultant is her role model, his opinion in incorporated into Louise's ideas of general practice. All her experience of GP at this stage of her career is similarly indirect, so she accepts the consultant's skill and knowledge are greater than that of local GPs who have referred patients to hospital. She is afraid of becoming that GP who is derided for their referrals:

> 'I am fairly sure that I would work [as a GP] in emergency at least one day a week. I just think I need that to keep my skills up and to keep my decision making up in terms of knowing who really needs to go to hospital and who doesn't.' (Louise)

For the first time, the question of what makes a good GP can be seen to differ between primary and secondary care. For Louise's consultant, being a good GP means not making work for the hospital. Within GP, it is a far more complex construct. The act of referral across the care interface occurs at a site of tension, and is a type of local contentious practice. GP trainees inadvertently become part of this practice, and their identities (the on-the-ground position of their current work placement and their early GP identity) end up in conflict. In contrast to Louise's acceptance, Emma again draws on her F2 experience to contest this hospital-centric view of GP work:

> 'People will say, that stupid GP has sent that patient up but I'm like, you don't understand what it's like sitting there and I will fight their corner and you don't understand what it's like sitting there and I think everybody should spend time in GP.' (Emma)

Emma is vociferous in her defence and frustration and again uses repetitive speech patterns to underline her point. Kerry and Clare, also with direct GP experience, both contest the same idea in similar ways:

'I think you have to do it [GP] to understand.' (Clare)

   'A lot of the time in A&E you do send them home, but you have the comfort of your bloods and your x-rays and you know you also have a senior there to also cast an eye over the patient. … I think everybody at some point should have to do, have some work in GP and A &E because I think no matter what specialty you go into it gives you the appreciation of first line medicine and what comes through … you sort of realise now that actually that's a GP who just couldn't send that person home.' (Kerry)

Clare recognises that understanding GP is related to on-the-ground practice in this setting, while Kerry uses her experience to inform her current work in A&E. She is able to pinpoint the differences between the two care settings, in particular, the availability of tests to mediate decision making and working with a team rather than autonomously.

Whatever their reaction to it, their experience of the longstanding primary-secondary care tension becomes an unavoidable part of the GP trainees' identities. Cultural norms and ideas of social positioning are passed down through everyday experience [7]. Unless historical inequalities and misunderstandings are corrected and contested, then they continue to be accepted as the status quo. Trainees are caught in the grip of these forces, and whether or not they can see a positive way out of it is largely down to how available other 'storylines' are to them. Within this small (non-statistical) sample, experience of working in primary care was a strong counter to negative positioning by hospital doctors. It allowed trainees access to an alternative narrative, and this seemed to improve their resilience to negative messages.

Conclusion

The primary-secondary care interface is a site of longstanding tension, which can be referred to in theoretical terms as enduring struggle. GP trainees are positioned right at the coalface, leaving them facing potential conflict through local contentious practice. They have to find a way to resolve this contradiction, either through accepting negative messages about GPs and by extension themselves, or by drawing on alternative narratives to contest such messages. Holland and Lave suggest that these sorts of interfaces are major sites for identity development, as people engage with social and cultural contexts to write their own stories [7].

The following chapter is a longitudinal case study of the last participant, Maria, who agreed to be interviewed three times over the course of her training: twice in hospital and once after her last move to the community.

REFERENCES

1. Miller KA, Boling B, Doyle DN. Emigrants and exiles: Irish cultures and Irish emigration to North America, 1790–1922. Ir Hist Stud [Internet]. 2016/07/28 ed. 1980;22(86):97–125. https://www.cambridge.org/core/article/emigrants-and-exiles-irish-cultures-and-irish-emigration-to-north-ame rica-1790-1922/9A3490AEF94062DA49D12B629BDCE0AB.
2. Goranson A, Sheeran P, Katz J, Gray K. Doctors are seen as godlike: moral typecasting in medicine. Soc Sci Med [Internet] 2020 Aug 1;258:113008. http://www.sciencedirect.com/science/article/pii/S0277953620302276.
3. Cameron A, Brangan E, Gabbay J, Klein JH, Pope C, Wye L. Discourses of joint commissioning. Health Soc Care Community [Internet]. 2018 Jan 1 [cited 2020 Dec 22];26(1):65–71. https://doi.org/10.1111/hsc.12462.
4. Norredam M, Album D. Review article: prestige and its significance for medical specialties and diseases. Scand J Public Health [Internet]. 2007 Dec 1 [cited 2020 Dec 22];35(6):655–661. https://doi.org/10.1080/14034940701362137.
5. Nic Craith M. Culture and identity politics in Northern Ireland. Basingstoke: Palgrave Macmillan; 2003.
6. Bennett D. Career choice in medicine [PhD thesis] [Internet]. Cork Open Research Archive; 2015. https://cora.ucc.ie/bitstream/handle/10468/2144/Deirdre%20Bennett%20PhD%20Thesis%20-%20Career%20Choice%20in%20MedicineFinalSubmitted.pdf?sequence=2&isAllowed=y.
7. Holland D, Lave J. History in person: enduring struggles, contentious practice, intimate identities. Santa Fe: School of American Research Press; 2001.
8. Hill E, Vaughan S, Hill E, Vaughan S. The only girl in the room: how paradigmatic trajectories deter female students from surgical careers. Med Educ. 2013;47(6):547–56.
9. Holland DC. Identity and agency in cultural worlds. Cambridge, MA: Harvard University Press; 1998.

CHAPTER 3

Maria's Narrative

Abstract This chapter builds on the phenomenological (lived experience) narratives of Chap. 2, this time focusing on the longitudinal progress of a single female GP trainee. Navigating different medical subcultures on clinical rotations, she can be seen to negotiate her overarching identity as a future GP alongside a pragmatic acceptance of her day-to-day position. Experience gained in general practice during the Foundation Scheme is seen to be fundamental to resolving the identity conflicts arising during the time in hospital placements.

Keywords GP • Identity • Postgraduate training • Medical education • Narrative analysis • NHS

In this chapter, Maria's narrative is presented over three interviews and two years of her training. Two interviews took place when she was in hospital and the last one when she had moved to the community as a GP the second year of specialty training (ST2) (following eighteen months based in hospitals). This adds a longitudinal aspect to the narratives given from participants in the last chapter, and allows a deeper look at the effects of paradigm conflict on individual identity and practice. The final move from a secondary to primary care base is a paradigm shift which brings about a transformation of Maria's professional self.

J. L. Johnston, *Conflict, Culture and Identity in GP Training*, https://doi.org/10.1007/978-981-19-2964-9_3

43

The idea of identities constantly changing over time is a central one in thinking about the conversation that takes place between individuals and their social and cultural contexts. French philosopher Paul Ricoeur, who was fascinated by how people use stories to reconstruct themselves over time, said that 'narrative identity takes place in the story's movement, in the dialectic between order and disorder' [1]. A dialectic is where two opposing ideas meet, and the clash between them can generate something new and useful. Ricouer is suggesting that sense of self is more about personal journey than it is about destination, incorporating our experiences, learning from them and being changed by them all the time.

This is an interesting idea in thinking about the journey of GP trainees as they pass through hospital training, where they are really just visiting, and into the world of primary care. All throughout this time, they compare their current work and identity with old versions of themselves, and with hopes and plans for the future. Maria reflects in her story on many of the same issues raised by other trainees in the last chapter, and is able to do so from a position of security at the end of her training. She uses her narrative to actively make sense of the more challenging experiences to date, in a way that integrates them into a coherent experience. In some ways, this is analogous to a patient's history, where illness and healthcare experience are integrated in a way that helps make sense of them. Maria moves between her past, present and future, sometimes returning to old stories with a new sense of meaning.

Maria started her hospital training with acute hospital (general) medicine, then moved on to work in psychiatry, paediatrics and then into GP. She worked in a large regional hospital in Derry/ Londonderry (the city is known as both, but is referred to from here onwards as Derry, the term that Maria uses), the second city of Northern Ireland, close to her home across the border with the Republic of Ireland in Donegal. Because she was speaking at multiple time points, her narrative is complex and not linear. For example, she talks a lot about working in general medicine, but little about her time in paediatrics. Her story is presented here in a narrative rather than a chronological way to stay close to her voice, and long extracts are used for the same reason. Within the 'big', overall story, there are lots of 'small stories' which she uses to build a picture of her working life and her professional self [2]. As in the previous chapter, she also links her professional identity with ideas of a future home life and personal identities such as motherhood.

The 'Home' Metaphor

The first interview took place about six weeks into the GP training scheme, and Maria had just finished a night shift in acute medicine. She was starting GP training directly from the foundation programme, during which she had had a GP placement which had been a very formative experience. The idea of home, both geographically and professionally, comes up again and again for her. As seen in the previous chapter, this has a special meaning on the island of Ireland given the long history of emigration. Maria had completed her medical school and foundation training in England, and recently returned to live in Donegal and work in nearby Derry. She therefore crossed the (invisible) Republic of Ireland/ Northern Ireland border every day. Here is Maria's introduction of herself:

'I am 26. I studied medicine in Norwich. I did my F1 and F2 in Manchester. But I am originally from [Co Donegal] so that's why I came back here. What else, erm ... before I started medicine, and during medicine I worked in an amusements. And coached football ... I was never good at football, my dad is a football coach for the Football Association of Ireland, and it was sort of compulsory to do it when I was younger. And then I was like, helped him and a method of income for us during the summer and he made us get our coaching badges, and that is pretty much what I did them for the rest of the summer. ... But it was good fun, and it was a reason to spend a weekend outside or a summer outside and it was a nice job and I like kids and it was working with kids and that was good. Erm—so I don't play it anymore, it was—now that I have a job that has a regular income I don't have to do it.'

While it might look like this is a bit of humorous small talk, Maria is actually offering a strong opening statement which links her home and work identities. She presents a strong and comfortable sense of belonging in her own context. Like Louise in the last chapter, she has moved away for a while and is now coming back home to settle into adult working life. At this point, she has accepted a GP training place in Derry knowing that it will bring her home to live and work, and she uses this information to frame all the subsequent conversation.

'When it came close to the time for closing applications I was just—I think I was in a period where I was homesick, so I was just like I am going to go home and I spoke to my parents and they were like, yeah great, yeah come home and I was like, okay fine. ... I moved from the Monday and started here on the Wednesday, but yeah it was quite a long drive (laughs). But my parents came over to get me, stayed for a couple of days in England, erm ... then we came back and as I say I am living with them now, erm ... and it's really nice there, like coming home to like a homemade dinner and it's good.'

Using humour and understatement is a way of underlining how important this decision was. She chose to situate her postgraduate training within her home context, making it much more likely that she would stay there for the long term. Connecting these two concepts of home and work makes Maria's story part of a master narrative of Irish emigration and return. This is a discourse which may also be familiar to medical graduates from other locations returning home after working abroad. GPs have the privilege of becoming embedded in communities which they serve. More than most specialties, GPs gain an insight into the lives and contexts of their patients, and may, like Maria, choose to share many of their patients' surrounding contexts. This link recurs throughout Maria's narrative and helps her to structure her story.

Like Niamh, for whom the decision to become a GP was related to her plans for a family, Maria finds a flexibility in GP than she perceives as absent in hospital training:

'Like obviously—life is important too, like I like that I don't have to work weekends if I don't want to and I don't have to do nights if I don't want to, like obviously if I wanted to do paediatrics or whatever you just—your life just, your work just has to fit around your life.'

In her need for good work-life balance, Maria is also subtly referring to her plans to become a parent in future. Once again, there is a background assumption that GP work is a more suitable choice for a woman. Maria's choice of a GP career is partially influenced by its flexibility, shorter training scheme and lack of mandatory out-of-hours commitment. This does not imply less commitment to her work, but a need to experience life as a whole which contests the traditional discourse of an almost priest-like commitment to medicine. Arguably, total commitment to career is a traditionally male privilege, with female narratives of work-life balance offering an important corollary to 'hero' narratives of medicine. Maria's story is the classic tale of homecoming expressed in two different ways, one literal and one metaphorical:

'So, in ten years' time I will hopefully be in Ireland again. As a GP partner somewhere, hopefully with a couple of kids. And a husband for the kids [laughs]. We had some motivational speaker lectures when I was an F2, this is a bit embarrassing, and he said just to have a plan, like a ten year plan and you should look at it, have it something that you can see so that it's reinforced every day that that's what I am working for. Plus, I like animals, and maybe like a little farm, but we will see.'

MOVING THROUGH TRAINING

Like Clare, Emma and Kerry, Maria draws on her F2 GP placement which was a formative part of her experience:

'It was meant to be a bit of a dossy [easy] job as an F2. … I didn't want to have lunchtimes free because I would have nothing to do with them, so when I started I said that I wanted to do everything that they were doing [the qualified GPs worked over lunch]. So I was doing all the, like, obviously it wasn't really like being a GP because I had 20 minute consultations [rather than the standard 10 minutes] and if I had any questions they [the GPs] were there, but I was busy all the time, it was really interesting, there were still children, I quite like obstetrics and I saw a few pregnant ladies … I just find it really interesting.'

The hegemonic position of secondary care is obvious here in the idea of GP F2 being easier than its hospital equivalent. Maria's own experiences are different, however, and sensitise her to the different paradigms of care. She enjoys the diversity of GP work and feels like part of a practice team. She also experiences good mentorship, one aspect of hospital posts which is often problematic for GP trainees, and so can learn within a safe and defined space. She is supported to 'try on' this identity and explore professional possibilities for herself. Back in hospital and having started her GP training scheme, she is still very influenced by her GP F2 rotation:

'It was just nice to like see somebody and be like, that continuity which you don't really get in hospital, because they come in again and they leave and you never see them again, or they might come again but you only see them for that sort of we will get you better and then get you out again.'

While she might not phrase it as such, Maria is expressing the value she places on the relational care that is central to GP. This aligns with her own values, and contrasts with what she perceives as an outcomes-based approach in hospital. She places herself confidently within the world of GP from early on, although she struggles to put her finger on exactly why:

'I just find it [GP] really interesting, and I don't like hospital medicine, I learned as an F1 that much … I think just, I don't know I have just never really—since I have been in—maybe it's just because I have been an F1 and an F2 and it's just been really stressful, I have never really sort of—I don't know. GP is going to be stressful. I don't know, I have just never really caught on, not caught onto it but it's never really caught onto me maybe I don't know. But nothing specific, nothing that I can say that is why I hate about, I don't hate it.'

Like other trainees, Maria understands competence in hospital medicine to be mediated through the performance of practical procedures. Here she reflects on her experiences in paediatrics as an F2:

'I think it was more just because I had done adult medicine for so long, and I was reasonably good you know like at procedures and knowing what is going on and not feeling out of my depth, and then I started paeds and felt out of my depth, couldn't get a cannula in for love nor money. And I just felt a bit like I am not good at this. And then—and it just—I don't know why I didn't—but I wasn't that—and again it was hospital medicine which I am not that fussed on either.'

This is one of the greatest challenges that GP trainees face while working in hospital—the constant rotations without being able to transfer skills. Hospital trainees in specialty training also face the challenge of multiple rotations between teams and units, but are at least able to carry their acquired expertise with them. Maria comments here on having got comfortable working in adult medicine and finding the move to paediatrics challenging. She experiences this as fundamental challenge to her sense of capability, rather than just a lack of experience.

For Maria, time spent in hospital is just a means to an end, with GP offering her an alternative and a way out of her sense of not belonging. As a GP trainee in hospital, she at least has a particular status and something to work towards:

'I knew this is what it was going to be like and I am happy enough in the job I'm in now, because it's only six months and I know it's not forever. And it's only a year in the hospital, which is doable. And then it's GP after that, so.'

The 'so' at the end of her story is a local expression which acts both as a full stop and conveys a sense of resignation. She finds the time in hospital challenging but accepts it is a means to an end and focuses on her end goal. GP is a kind of promised land at the end of a difficult journey.

By the time of her second interview, Maria has moved into working in psychiatry, with very different working practices from acute medicine. Even the physical space is different, as she is now working in a separate mental health facility. Maria feels closer to GP as she gets to work with the primary care liaison team and spends most of her time in outpatient clinics. She is able to lift her head from just getting through and think about herself as a GP in the near future:

'You know I will have finished hospital medicine in another—10 months. And then it will—I have a year and a half in GP in then that's me, I'm a GP. I don't know whether I will be ready at that stage. … I think because I am in clinics now and it's all outpatient I feel a bit more like I am moving towards GP than I did when I was in medicine. But I still don't feel like I am a GP and there is not the same, I don't feel like there is the same responsibility as if—do you know if I say, right I have changed this person's medicine I don't think I need to be involved anymore, back to the GP. You can't do that when you are a GP because you are back to the GP. There is no getting away from it.'

Maria hits on a fundamental truth here. The flip side of being an autonomous practitioner is accepting final responsibility for patient care. Because GP training is so relatively short, she will experience this responsibility much earlier than her peers in hospital specialty training. For the first time, she is expressing some concern about whether she will be prepared enough for such a big transition. She has a strong identity as a GP trainee in hospital but recognises that this will soon shift to a new identity, as a GP trainee in the community.

By the time she moves from psychiatry to her final hospital post (paediatrics, for the second time as she also worked there in F2), the end is in sight. This last post in hospital serves a functional purpose but she finds it unremarkable:

'I'd done four months of paeds before [in F2] and I enjoyed that too like, before I decided that I wanted to do GP I was going to do paediatrics, but then I did GP and decided, oh I'm doing that instead. So I like paediatrics but working in it the first time sort of reinforced that I didn't want to do it. And I enjoyed it again this time but it is just—I suppose it's the same as like it's just really understaffed and really busy and ... but it was still an enjoyable job.'

Maria notes the importance of work experience here—she discounted a paediatric career after working there in F2. All through her reflections on working in hospital, Maria works hard to cast even more challenging experiences in a positive light. Finally, though, when she makes the big move into general practice after eighteen months and feels she has a bit more freedom to reflect on the difficulties:

'I was delighted to get finished with the hospital ... I finished my last day in paediatrics—was on call, and apparently they've never seen anybody so giddy! It was just like I'll do whatever you want, doesn't matter because I'll never see you again. And it's been really nice because I've been—this practice is really nice and all the GPs have been sound [very friendly] and really helpful. And yeah it's been nice.'

There is a strong sense of release in this small story of drawing a line and moving forward. There is little integration between hospital and community—Maria crosses the line and that is the end of her association with hospital work. She is really coming into her own now and being received into her own community, rather than constantly being on the edge of someone else's. In one sense, this is where the real business of situated learning and translation of hospital-acquired skills will begin.

EDUCATION VERSUS SERVICE PROVISION

When she was in hospital, Maria drew on her F2 GP experience, and as a GP trainee in the community, she reflects her hospital experience. She worries that not having done a hospital placement in gynaecology will put her at a disadvantage:

'I haven't had any experience in [gynae], well I've had loads of experience since I've come here ... but I haven't got any proper obs & gynae training ... it's not, like, I don't feel that confident with it and I feel like as a

female GP I should be confident in obs and gynae. But then I suppose—
there's going to be others who haven't done paeds and they won't feel—
whereas I'm quite confident, reasonably confident with paeds, and I suppose
it just will come … I have picked up loads since I've been here even but I
would've—for starting this job I would've felt more comfortable if I've
done a little bit of gynae etc. I don't think I've done anything dangerous—
or, and it's fine because [her trainer] is downstairs so like I've got back up
from that point of view.'

In this narrative not only is there a worry about wanting to be safe in
her autonomous practice, but also an internalisation of the hospital being
the site of 'excellent' medical education. As discussed in Chap. 1, this is a
deep-rooted discourse which can be traced back to Osler [3]. Despite
'loads of experience' of managing gynaecology issues in primary care,
Maria is aware that this is not formalised education and is therefore concerned that it may not count. She is engaged in on-the-job workplace
learning, and is quickly filling knowledge gaps with workplace learning
and the help of her supportive trainer.

Despite her worries about missing out on hospital training, there is an
evident conflict as she is disparaging about the educational value of some
of her hospital posts:

'Mostly, I find generally when you are in hospital it's mostly service provision, maybe that's why I have not liked hospital medicine, because like I see
the patients on the ward round but I don't do that much with them on my
day job, I don't get to speak that much to them really, unless I need to put
a cannula in or something. So there is not—unless somebody gets sick I
don't really review anybody it's just the ward round. And then you are just
doing jobs and ordering scans and chasing scans and it's all sort of a bit, not
boring, boring is not the right word but I just feel a bit like—a service
provider.'

Maria is in a position lacking in agency as a junior medical doctor, and
instead is required to carry out decisions made by more senior doctors.
The work is repetitive, highlighted with the rhythm and choice of words
in the phrase 'just doing jobs and ordering scans and chasing scans [get-
ting results].' The 'jobs' she refers to in this context mean routine ward
work such as taking bloods, siting cannulas and ordering radiology tests.
Unfortunately, Maria is having the same experience as her specialty peers,
based on a tight hierarchy and cultural norms within acute hospital

medicine. This time spent doing menial work is, even in the present day, considered something of a rite of passage. The ward round takes on a slightly theatrical aspect in which the consultant is the chief player:

> 'I understand we all have to do it and you wouldn't expect a consultant to be running around, because they have done it before and they have come through that and that's fine and I understand that, but it's just not that interesting ... I think mostly, like I don't really mind coming in early and staying late and stuff if people are sick and things need done, but I just don't like all the service provision.'

There is quite a contrast here with the type of workplace learning Maria had experience of in F2 as a GP and then encounters again as an ST2. As a very junior GP F2, she engaged fully in the work of the GP practice rather than being assigned different menial work. After moving to a community ST2 post, Maria reflects back on her hospital experiences from her current viewpoint in general practice:

> 'When you're in hospital it's sort of like—it's sort of like a tick box exercise almost, like you're seeing the patient, you know somebody's coming after you, you know there's like certain questions, obviously there's still certain questions you need to ask and there's, you're just filling out a proforma, presenting complaint, history of presenting complaint da da da da da—and it's like obviously you've got more time to spend with them, and you ask about loads of random things that I probably wouldn't ask about any more—just, unless I thought it was—necessary, and it's just, I don't know sometimes people come in and I feel like it's a bit more of a chat here, whereas in hospital I was like, it's very much you're just going in and being like right, I need to get through this proforma of what I need to ask you and then I'm going to examine you and then I'll see you later.'

A contrast is drawn here between the different approaches to history-taking, and indeed different approaches to the whole consultation within primary and secondary care paradigms. Much undergraduate and hospital training utilises a systems-based approach, where a standard format covering each body system is used with every patient history. This can sometimes end with the doctor asking about irrelevancies and long lists of negatives ('loads of random things that I probably wouldn't ask about anymore.') In hospital, medical hierarchy is reinforced through this practice, in which she prepares the ground for a senior doctor to make decisions. General practice utilises a problem-based (targeted) history instead. Maria's language is also suggestive of the pervasive efficiency discourse in healthcare, through the phrases 'tick-box exercise,' 'da da da da' and 'I need to get through this.' Signing off her narrative, Maria's 'see you later' is a little sarcastic, underscoring her transient encounters with patients in hospital.

Given that she finds in-hours work dull in medicine, Maria welcomes on-call work because she can be more autonomous. She can think and act independently and, like Laura, is quick to underline her own capacity in dealing with emergencies in hospital:

> 'So like, I like seeing the patient for the first time and doing the management plan or whatever you are going to do, erm … and I don't mind seeing really sick patients, I am not, like I don't think that I perform badly under pressure or anything. I think I perform quite well under pressure, but—so I liked it from that point of view, erm … but you tended not to—d'you know you tended not to see those patients again and when you admit them they go to whatever ward they go to and you never really see them again and then you go back to your own ward and you just do jobs.'

There is a sense of dull inevitability to Maria's abrupt conclusion that she just goes back to do 'jobs' after these brief encounters. Yet in feeling able to manage sick hospital patients on her own, there is a rare chance to express a sense of self as a doctor. In technical terms, she finds a space for agency [4] in the breaks from routine work. Spending half her training time in hospital, Maria joins the other trainees in constantly juggling her imagined future self in GP and her current, on the ground, and often subordinate position in hospital. Particularly in acute medicine, she feels she is primarily there as a service doctor, and feels compressed by this role.

AT THE COALFACE OF PARADIGM CONFLICT

As other trainees were in the previous chapter, Maria is embroiled in the longstanding conflict between primary and secondary care. This is an inevitable consequence of training for GP in an environment where secondary care retains a hegemonic position. In other words, the idea of secondary care as 'better' has become taken for granted and normalised over time. Education is one key process by which this power imbalance is maintained; trainees have a choice to either accept inferior positioning, aligning themselves with the taken-for-granted attitude, or to challenge it. It has been well documented here and elsewhere that GP trainees in hospital are often subject to negative messages about their choice. Maria has similar experiences, whereby she is drawn into the conflict by more senior hospital doctors. She relates this conversation as an F2 in paediatrics:

> 'And I remember when I was doing … like before I started GP training but I had already applied to GP, I was on paediatrics and the consultant, I was in clinic with the consultant and I was just sitting in and I wasn't seeing patients, it was the first one I think and then she said, she was doing some teaching and then she said what have you applied for and I said GP, and she said oh this is sort of a waste of my time then, and I was like I can't believe you just said that [laughs]. I just kept stum [quiet] … it's just sort of, I don't know I suppose they sort of think people have gone into GP it's a bit of a cop out almost. I don't feel that it's a cop out but they seem to [laughs].'

Maria's laughter takes some of the sting out of this story, but it is obvious that she found this exchange difficult. The senior doctor shows an overt lack of respect for Maria and for GP work in general. The hierarchy between them makes it difficult for Maria to challenge this outright, but it causes her to consider her career decision. A second similar experience occurred during her GP hospital training:

> 'I find, and it sort of annoys me, like say for example, this—one of the consultants who is really nice and I got on really well with, the first time I met him we were going round on the ward round and he said, he asked me what I was doing and I said I was a GP trainee. And he said, oh that's a shame you would be good enough to be a hospital doctor. And I was like does that mean that people who aren't good go into GP?! I am not sure that that is really a compliment that you have just given me.'

Of the two, this interaction is less aggressive but has potential to be even more damaging as a result of their positive relationship and his role as a mentor. He positions Maria as underselling herself with her commitment to GP, the subtext of which is that she could achieve more as a hospital doctor. Both these consultants perpetuate longstanding inequality, and both play on the power structures of hospital in a way which makes it difficult for Maria to contest their views.

'It doesn't make me think, oh I should have done hospital medicine instead. It just makes me think that they have a silly opinion about—not a silly opinion that's not the right word, but—probably the wrong opinion (laughs) about what—like being a GP is. But then like a lot of them will say that, but then they will be the first to turn around and say, there are plenty of good GPs out there who make our work a lot easier.'

Despite contesting such a negative position for herself, in struggling to be fair, Maria ventriloquises the consultant's authoritative voice at the end. The idea of a 'good GP' as a GP who makes life easier for hospital was introduced in the last chapter. GP work is assumed to be 'secondary care lite'—a less complex, more distilled down version of hospital work.

In the previous chapter, it was seen that during their training time in hospital, an important means of contesting trainees' negative position in hospital was by building an alternative community of practice. This is also true for Maria. Although trainees were not often in a position to directly defend negative messages, they found some relief in connecting with other GP trainees working in different parts of the hospital. GP trainees in hospital can be considered marginal to a traditional community of practice, for example, in cardiology or paediatrics. They were able to construct, however, an alternative based on the shared practices of learning to become GPs while managing day-to-day hospital work. They were connected first and foremost by a sense of *not* belonging. Like her peers in the previous chapter, Maria finds that core GP training sessions—usually a half-day release once a month—give her important opportunities, both for networking and constructing a place for herself in the world of GP.

'…and then like we've done presentations on, erm … prescribing and adverse incidents in prescribing and sort of generic prescribing and things like that. Erm … and it's all probably things that I don't remember that much about now do you know like I had the lecture and found it interesting at the time and now I don't remember that much. … Probably not so much [useful] for hospital, but it's things like when we did the prescribing, erm … and they were saying about generic prescribing and looking at costs and practice costs and things like that, they did like a, we had a talk from a pharmacist, erm … on sort of reducing certain types of prescribing because it costs the practice too much and benefit analysis for the patient and things like that. Which you don't have to do at all in hospital and you just try what you are told or what you fancy, not what you fancy but … and you don't think about costs at all and it sort of makes you think about why am I pre-scribing this then rather than a different type of thing.'

Speaking here in her last interview, while working in a GP practice, Maria finds it difficult to remember the detail of what content was covered in past core days. What has stuck is not the content but a sense of how important it was to explore beyond the day-to-day work of the hospital. Generic prescribing and cost-benefit analysis might not sound attention-grabbing, but had the attraction of being both completely foreign to hospital and familiar to GP work. Prescribing practice, like so many other aspects, varies enormously between primary and secondary care. Talking about artefacts of GP like prescribing, consulting or significant event analysis allowed GP trainees in hospital to practise their community identities and renew their sense of commitment to this future. Here is Maria speaking from an earlier interview in a hospital post:

'So last week or was it the last one we had, it wasn't last week, erm … was on consultation skills and you just went through the different types of consultation skills, because I only knew about the Calgary Cambridge because that's what I learnt about in medical school and I didn't know that there was any other type of consultation skill, except that [GP] had mentioned something, like a comment on my portfolio and I thought I should look that up and didn't. Erm … and he was talking about, I have forgotten them all now … erm … Neighbour. And it was really interesting and he sort of mentioned a few books, erm … that we should look at.'

Roger Neighbour is a legendary authority on the consultation in GP circles [5]. This is new information for Maria, and she is interested without really understanding its significance yet. Maria uses this reference to make a claim on a new, community-based GP identity.

This, together with other mediators such as problem-based consulting, help Maria to construct a grounded idea of her future professional self.

Core education days were an essential lifeline to general practice from hospital placements for the trainees. Working in her final hospital post, in paediatrics, Maria finds herself isolated without these basic peer contacts. A small number of day release clinics with her GP supervisor have to fill the gap left.

'There was none [core GP days] when I was in that six months in hospital which was a bit sort of, not tough, tough's not the right word but—you just, you don't really see anybody … it was just nice to sort of keep it relevant to—because when you're in six months in hospital and you're not really thinking about GP, you come here, I came here three times, maybe four times just to sort of see my trainer and have a chat and I think I did a couple of sort of clinics with him, and that was it but you sort of, I don't know, I feel like you could lose track of what you're supposed to be doing and you're just concentrating on getting through paeds … so you lose track of the fact that you're a GP trainee and not—not a paediatric trainee.'

Just as the end is in sight, Maria starts to worry about her GP identity slipping away. This illustrates the pressure that GP trainees are under in hospital. They are often perceived as lower status, but yet do not benefit from being different. In these trainees' experiences, they are there primarily to do the service work of any other junior doctor from any other training scheme. Minimal attention is paid to their particular needs during this period.

GETTING TO KNOW HERSELF AS A GP

In Maria's narrative, a clear difference emerges in the identity and experience of hospital- and community-based GP trainees; the former working hard to connect to the GP world, and the latter joining a better recognised model of a community of practice. This is an under-recognised subtlety with important pedagogical implications. When Maria makes her final move into community during her ST2 year, she starts a completely new journey of identity and learning. Here, she reviews her experiences to date:

'But it's just I never really thought about doing anything else, like I don't ever really remember wanting to be anything but a doctor and I don't think I ever really thought about what it was going to be like or how hard it would be or, do you know I think I was just like I'm going to be a doctor and that's what I'm going to do … and that was it and I got into it and I enjoyed it thank God, and it worked out ok but I … I don't think I thought about what was important to me. … I think I'm probably, well I don't think I'm a diff—I don't know … obviously I've gone from being seventeen to twenty seven and I'm different, but I think I'd have become more like responsible anyway because you're going from seventeen to twenty seven em but yeah I don't know.'

In ten years, she has gone from being a medical student in England to being a qualified doctor working as a GP trainee in Derry, Northern Ireland. At each stage, she has had to imagine a future for herself in order to make that future happen. She is confident she has found her niche, after completing the two-year foundation programme and another eighteen months in hospital. During this time, her relationships with both primary and secondary care paradigms evolve. She now has to imagine how she wants her life and work to look as an independent, fully qualified GP.

As she noted earlier, there is a significant difference in the style of consulting between hospital and GP practice. Maria evolves her own style of consulting to encompass relational and longitudinal care, providing a valuable metaphor for the change in her practice and identity:

> 'You know that you're probably going to see them again and you don't have to do everything right now and—I think I'm slightly less formal than I used to be, just in terms of patients coming in and having a bit of a chat rather than—whereas before when I was in hospital and when I was in GP previously I was just a bit like, I'm a doctor, d'you know, what am I doing for you and then—see you later, and that was it whereas, I don't know, like patients coming in and they like tell me about their holidays and things ... whereas before I would've been like, (taps fingers) this isn't relevant ... when you're in hospital you're just sort of constantly having other things and like I would've, I wouldn't have been like we are not talking about your holiday but I would've quickly—moved that conversation on ... whereas now I'm just a bit like oh right yeah that's really nice tell me about your holiday.'

Once again, efficiency discourse is present in the narrative. While it would be disingenuous to suggest this discourse is not also at play in primary care settings, Maria has a key realisation: the holiday chat is not meaningless time-wasting, but is a building block in an important therapeutic relationship.

In her final interview, Maria draws her past, present and future together. She returns again to the theme of home in expressing her hope for the future:

> 'So yeah the plan at the minute is probably just to ... locum for a couple of years, go on holidays and then try and get a, try and get a partnership ... hopefully [in] Derry—just because like I only live down the road and like I'm from [Donegal] and everyone, all my sort of family and stuff is down

there and obviously my partner's down there and so yeah ... hopefully stay here in Derry, it's just really handy for me.'

CONCLUSION

This chapter has followed Maria's story as she dealt with challenging aspects of hospital training and moved on into the community. This allowed a deeper and more nuanced analysis of the issues which arose in the last chapter. Maria's story also forms a case study of the transition from hospital to community-based GP training, with the associated shifts in practice and identity.

Throughout, the longstanding paradigm conflict and inequality form a background to her experiences. Wider issues of hierarchy and pedagogy in hospital settings are also raised. In the next two chapters, these issues are explored and radical changes to the structures of GP training are suggested.

REFERENCES

1. Ricoeur P. Reflections on a new ethos for Europe. In: Paul Ricoeur: the hermeneutics of action. London: Sage; 1996.
2. Bamberg M. Stories: big or small: why do we care? Narrat Enq. 2006;16(1):139–47.
3. Bliss M. William Osler: a life in medicine. Toronto: University of Toronto Press; 1999.
4. Holland DC. Identity and agency in cultural worlds. Cambridge, MA: Harvard University Press; 1998.
5. Neighbour R. The inner consultation. Lancaster: MTP Press; 1987.

CHAPTER 4

Paradigms in Conflict

Abstract This chapter pulls together the narratives of lived experience of Chaps. 2 and 3, integrating them with other empirical and theoretical perspectives to define a new concept of the *primary care paradigm*—a distinct set of practices underpinned by its own philosophy and structures, and with a separate pedagogy. The philosophical standpoint of primary care is outlined in terms of its ontology, epistemology and axiology, and a practitioner identity outlined which utilises these coherently in everyday work, including at the primary care interface.

Keywords Primary care • Paradigms • NHS • GP • Identity • NHS

In this chapter, trainee narratives are drawn together with other empirical literature and theoretical concepts. The primary care paradigm is defined in terms of its philosophy and practice, and questions of power and identity are explored through the concept of *paradigm conflict*. The pedagogical impact of this enduring struggle is explored in terms of its impact on both GP trainees and experienced practitioners. In the next chapter, suggestions are made for impact on policy and practice.

© The Author(s), under exclusive license to Springer Nature   61
Singapore Pte Ltd. 2022
J. L. Johnston, *Conflict, Culture and Identity in GP Training*,
https://doi.org/10.1007/978-981-19-2964-9_4

THEORISING THE PRIMARY CARE PARADIGM

A paradigm is a coherent set of assumptions about how the world works that colour human experience [1]. Primary and secondary care both fulfil this definition, with differences which are philosophical, structural and practical, culminating in two different ways of 'doing' medicine. Primary care is not classically recognised as a separate entity, but as a medical specialty—a subsection of the profession as a whole. Because of the hegemonic position of secondary care, it is easy to overlook just how different primary care is, making it easily misunderstood as an inferior copy of hospital practice. It can be understood to have a separate *ontology, epistemology* and *axiology*. These philosophical terms refer respectively to how GPs construct the nature of their professional realities, their knowledge and skills, and their underpinning values. All are described below.

Commitment to Generalism

Medicine in general practice is based on relational care offered via longitudinal relationships with patients. It is a truism to say that GPs treat people, while specialists treat diseases, but general practice is certainly predicated on the idea of a patient-centred physician, who works longitudinally with patients across their lifespan [2]. The traditional longitudinal model is a pillar of general practice, exemplifying the NHS mantra of cradle-to-grave. In the UK, GPs retain a strong commitment to their generalist status in the face of increasing subspecialisation and silo models of secondary care [3]. Practice is defined by breadth, although some GPs also choose to acquire in-depth knowledge and skills in an area of special interest. Hospital generalism is, by contrast, a rarity, having little currency in the hospital discourse which prioritises subspecialisation. As a result, GPs have an overview of patients' health and care which is important in detecting conflicting treatments and preventing over-diagnosis [4].

Complexity and Uncertainty

The breadth of practice and the primary care nature of GP work means that undifferentiated illness must be routinely managed. The fine balance of risk must be assessed for each consultation, meaning that *uncertainty* and *complexity* are defining features of the primary care paradigm [5]. These are skills which are taught under close supervision and assessed during professional GP exams [6]. In comparison, hospital patients will often have been triaged via their GP and have at least an early diagnosis made. In secondary care, practice is not about tolerating uncertainty but about eliminating it, usually through the use of tests [7].

The GP Consultation

The consultation is the primary building block of the doctor-patient relationship in primary care. It is the most important mediator of GP identity, and is widely taught and assessed in detail during GP training [6]. Research into the consultation has led to the development and integration of *consultation models*, which explicitly recognise the social work undertaken in consultations and their therapeutic potential.

One of the most influential consultation theorists is Michael Balint. His 1962 concept of the 'doctor as drug' recognises the dialogic nature of the primary care doctor-patient relationship. Balint noted doctors' 'apostolic function'—a tendency to form fixed beliefs about how patients should behave, which might reduce the therapeutic value of the relationship. He noted that not only does the clinician have feelings towards the patient, but also that these feelings should be processed through regular reflexive practice. If managed well, longstanding therapeutic relationships can be used to build a store of trust and goodwill between the patient and clinician. This 'mutual investment fund' can be drawn upon to encourage concordance with treatment, try new forms of management or see the relationship through difficult circumstances [8].

Other models have been integrated over years. Consulting has moved from a basic understanding of Maslow's hierarchy of needs [9], through Berne's transactional analysis [10], and multiple models which dissect the consultation into constituent parts (Byrne and Long [11], Stott and Davis [12], Pendleton [13]). One of the most influential contemporary theorists is Roger Neighbour, mentioned by Maria in the preceding chapter, whose key contributions include the concepts of safety netting and housekeeping; the former leaves the door open for patients to come back, and the latter means consciously moving on from the previous consultation to focus on the current one [14].

In primary care, history-taking moves to an integrated and problem-based style. The central position of the patient is respected with an emphasis on shared discovery and decision-making. Patients by and large wear their normal daytime clothes and attend a GP surgery within their own community. By contrast, in hospital, sick adult in-patients are likely to wear similar night clothes, lie in similar beds and become surrounded by medical technology. Patients can easily appear disembodied, making the classic objectification trap 'the chest infection in bed 6' (rather than 'Mrs Smith with the chest infection in bed 6') easier to fall into. In communities, by contrast, accrued contextual information makes it more difficult to separate patients from their personhood.

With its holistic approach and engagement in dialogue, the modern GP consultation can be seen as a rejection of a purely biomedical model and the clinical gaze; the latter is a way of being which affords power to the scientific and technological expertise of the clinician [15]. The body is seen as separate from the mind (*dualism*) and as a machine which is fixable like any other. The patient's own illness experience and narrative are discounted as unreliable, so that they occupy a subordinate and objectified position within the relationship.

In contesting the clinical gaze, both at individual and structural levels, the GP consultation becomes an *epistemological act*. Through this central activity, GP doctors come to know themselves and to engage in this particular way of knowing and practising medicine. General practice can be characterised as having a *narrative epistemology and ontology*, based on the exchange of stories (receiving histories, giving information and participating in shared decision-making).

The axiology of primary care is congruent with the rest of its philosophy. Professional values encompass community-based, person-oriented, multidisciplinary and longitudinal care. GPs are important advocates for their patients and wider population-level public health [4]. This advocacy ranges from individual issues, such as managing refused secondary care referrals, to a broader social justice agenda addressing social determinants of health. Prominent GP, Iona Heath, has characterised the primary care consultation as integrating 'the human experience of suffering and the paradigms of scientific medicine, with the general practitioner acting as an interpreter at the boundary between illness and disease, and a witness to suffering' [16].

GP and Hospital Consultations as Speech Genres

Consultations involve complex social actions mediated by particular forms of language use. As seen in Chap. 1, language not only represents, but also constructs meaning [17]. This is the source of the power within the consultation to change 'hard' health outcomes through a dialogic relationship with the patient.

The difference in primary and secondary care consultations is a discriminator of each paradigm, and can be understood as two different *speech genres*. These are mutually agreed conversational shortcuts, which are socioculturally situated. Use of a speech genre has a particular social meaning, and often means the speaker is claiming an identity as part of a particular group [17].

Given the centrality of the consultation in the world of GP, speech genres are one of the most important cultural artefacts. GPs no longer wear white coats and do not often wear a stethoscope round their necks, both material symbols used by other medical groups, but their particular genre of consultation is distinctive. Within the narratives, trainees use both hospital and GP genres to situate themselves and their work. For example, in Laura's story, her manner of talking about knee joint aspiration is a claim to belonging in hospital, and also showed some discomfort with her fledgling GP identity. She uses phrasing and medical jargon in keeping with hospital speech genres:

> 'Oh you're just a GP—I'm like, well no actually. Do you know if you want me to stick a needle in that knee I will, you know this isn't just something just for the medical trainees. Just cause I want to be a GP. All the regs and stuff are like, you're just a GP. It's like, not just!' (Laura)

On the other hand, her friend, Emma, with whom she was interviewed, has a strong connection to her GP self and has a different way of speaking about her experiences:

> 'People will say, that stupid GP has sent that patient up but I'm like, you don't understand what it's like sitting there and I will fight their corner and you don't understand what it's like sitting there and I think everybody should spend time in GP.' (Emma)

In Chap. 3, Maria's shift in identity is personified by the change in her consultation style after moving to the community:

> 'You know that you're probably going to see them again and you don't have to do everything right now and—I think I'm slightly less formal than I used to be, just in terms of patients coming in and having a bit of a chat rather than—whereas before when I was in hospital and when I was in GP previously I was just a bit like, I'm a doctor, d'you know, what am I doing for you and then—see you later, and that was it whereas, I don't know, like

patients coming in and they like tell me about their holidays and things ... whereas before I would've been like, (taps fingers) this isn't relevant ... when you're in hospital you're just sort of constantly having other things and like I would've, I wouldn't have been like we are not talking about your holiday but I would've quickly—moved that conversation on ... whereas now I'm just a bit like oh right yeah that's really nice tell me about your holiday.' (Maria)

Primary and secondary care genres can be seen to be defining features of each paradigm, discursively constructing medical practice and therefore identity.

Local Contentious Practice

As seen in Chaps. 2 and 3, the historical construction of primary care's lower status continues to play out within present-day cultural and social norms. Discourses of power are constructed on older, historical discourses and unless they are contested, they are passed down through generations [18]. Education is a vital means by which this happens [19].

At the heart of the paradigm conflict is lack of understanding in secondary care of the work of primary care as different in philosophy, identity and practice. Inevitably, hospital-based GP trainees find themselves positioned at this interface. Because of their greater exposure to it, and its hegemonic position as of higher status, hospital medicine become the 'baseline' in figuring the world of medicine. In other words, secondary care becomes the default through taken-for-granted assumptions, and GP trainees have to figure their identity against this. Working in hospitals but 'belonging' to general practice, they are inadvertently drawn into local contentious practice (the everyday activities that perpetuate the conflict).

Some of the clearest examples of local contentious practice are at the points where patients move from primary to secondary care and back again: that is, admission to and discharge from hospital. The primary-secondary care interface is a literal as well as theoretical boundary, and an acknowledged risk to patient safety in part because of the different professional practices on either side [20]. As was seen in the narratives, a 'good GP' was figured as being a GP who did not refer a lot of work to hospital. Yet this view is based on a profound lack of understanding of the primary care paradigm, with its management of uncertainty and risk.

At the other end, discharge letters are a chronic point of tension. These are traditionally completed by the most junior doctor on the team, with little awareness of what information the primary care physician might require. In recent years, patient safety initiatives, such as pharmacist reviews of discharge letters, have greatly improved medication safety. Other important information, however, such as whether follow up will be arranged and actions needed by the GP, remain open to poor communication. Legendary amongst GPs are the phrases 'GP to action' and 'GP to chase,', fraught as they are with assumptions about hierarchy and the relevance of secondary care models to primary care work [21].

WIDER IMPACTS

Longstanding paradigm conflict has two important impacts, on the professional development of individual trainees and on the conflict itself. The inferior position often afforded to hospital GP trainees, and the overt negative messages they receive, make the paradigm conflict a part of their developing identity. In other words, trainees' experiences perpetuate the conflict. Many of the doctors who are responsible for negative messaging are in a position of authority, with a mentoring relationship to the GP trainee who therefore finds it difficult to avoid or contest the conflict.

Coming to some accommodation with this inherent contradiction is an indispensable part of identity building. For the trainees who had done F2 GP placements (Clare, Kerry, Maria and Emma), this was a strong protective factor. Their experience allowed them to figure a realistic picture of the world of GP and their future place in it. They drew on this time while working in hospital, both to translate the work to something of use for their GP future, and as a form of resistance against negative positioning.

For the trainees without direct experience of general practice, it was much harder to counter negative attitudes. Three of the four had come to GP training after leaving hospital specialty training programmes, and the fourth had accepted a place in training as a back-up when she was not offered her first choice. Without direct experience, the picture they painted of themselves as GPs was drawn simply as an alternative to themselves as hospital doctors. This is a risky approach, because they may not fully understand the primary care paradigm themselves, and so are entering GP training blindly. These trainees have made particularly high stakes decisions, and so are in a more vulnerable position.

A further risk for all trainees is the immersive and relatively long nature of hospital-based GP training, which carries a risk of forgetting why they are there in the first place. Constant conflict from low-level negative positioning carries a risk of undermining their GP identities to the extent they leave training. Trainees were aware of this and consciously stayed close to their GP selves:

> 'I don't feel like I am a psychiatrist, sometimes I feel like I am pretending to be a psychiatrist … I think you have to remind yourself you are a GP trainee.' (Clare)
> 'I think knowing in the end that you are a generalist and not a specialist of anything that you see or come across now … you just have to keep that mindset in the days of A&E when it's, yeah you're feeling a bit down with it all.' (Kerry)

'BIG' DISCOURSES AND PARADIGM CONFLICT

All social life is marked by the 'big divisions' [22]. While the main focus here is on how language is used between people at the level of everyday social interactions, these take place against unavoidable large-scale discourses of power.

Healthcare as Industry

Within the contemporary NHS, discourses of efficiency, accountability and neoliberalism are prevalent [23–25]. Inevitably, junior doctors will find themselves part of a healthcare system which is itself engaged in an enduring struggle between two ideologies: the socialised healthcare foundations of the NHS, and free-market forces reflected in governmental cuts and a drive towards private medical provision [26–28]. This rhetoric is particularly obvious in Louise and David's narratives, both of whom had experience of other countries' healthcare systems and of other specialty training programmes. Louise's narrative is marked throughout by *decisiveness*, David's by *efficiency*. Both reference a dominant political discourse prioritising throughput and efficient use of services in an analogy to industry [24, 28, 29].

As seen in the narratives, efficiency discourse can profoundly suppress the voice of patients, and so is in conflict with fundamental tenets of general practice. While Maria learned to measure her own clinical competence in terms of speed and quantity as a junior doctor in acute medicine, she was also aware of a contradiction. Her phrase 'see you later' was delivered sarcastically, subtly expressing her discomfort at the compromises she felt forced to make in terms of patient care:

'...it's very much you're just going in and being like right, I need to get through this proforma of what I need to ask you and then I'm going to examine you and then I'll see you later.' (Maria)

Clare also refers to the efficiency discourse, and is both conscious and critical of it, suggesting that person-centred care should be secondary to throughput and efficiency.

Clare figures general practice as a way to swap forced efficiency for greater autonomy and patient-centeredness:

'There is a lot of pressure from bed managers and different things in hospitals that you just sometimes think that the patient's best interests aren't being put to the forefront. Whereas I don't know in GP you can kind of control that a little bit more.' (Clare)

General practice is at the sharp end of austerity and reductions in public sector funding, because political changes are inevitably played out in the theatre of available resources and enforced working patterns. GPs must reconcile this political aspect of practice with their ideals and hopes for the future. Choosing a career in general practice means finding a way to accommodate the mundane daily practices of the job within the political landscape.

GP as Gendered Practice

The intersection of gender with professional identity was perhaps inevitable given the largely female sample. It is most obvious in Niamh's story: like many other women working in surgery, she found herself positioned as an outsider in a male-dominated specialty [30, 31]. Her figured identity as a surgeon could not be reconciled with her figured identity as a potential future parent. Chen et al's study of surgical residents' experience of life events such as parenthood confirms Niamh's perception that there is less support available to female surgeons [32]. This was a significant part of self-building for her, motivating her to leave surgical training and to enter GP training. Because general practice offers a shorter period of training, no out-of-hours commitment, and flexibility with in-hours work [33], there is a still a commonly held belief within the medical community that it is a particularly suitable career choice for a woman [34]. This is built on layers of assumptions about primary care work and women's aspirations to having a family, while simultaneously discounting male doctors' parenthood. General practice is not often recognised as a gendered specialty in the same way as, for example, surgery, but is subject to gendering [35]. This may contribute to its perceived lack of prestige from within hospital. For female trainees in particular, the intersection of these assumptions with professional identity is so embedded within practice that it becomes difficult to see unless explicitly looked for [36].

Power Structures as Processes

Just like person-to-person interactions, large-scale discourses are socially constructed. At times, these power relations can become taken for granted, but they interact with other aspects of identity to influence the development of professional self.

It is helpful and important to realise that power structures are the result of human processes, not set in stone [18]. All social activity, including that at work, either upholds power structures, hierarchies and inequalities, or contests them. This is often done through talk in the smallest of ways. Recognising the influence of these forces opens up the possibility of change.

In the final chapter, issues of pedagogy within GP training are addressed, drawing on theoretical perspectives from Freire and Gramsci. Radical suggestions to the policy and practice of GP education are suggested to positively impact identities, and in turn retention and recruitment.

REFERENCES

1. Kuhn TS. The structure of scientific revolutions. Chicago: University of Chicago Press; 1962.
2. Simon C, Everitt H, van Dorp F, Burkes M. Oxford handbook of general practice. Oxford: Oxford University Press; 2014.
3. Leinster S. Training medical practitioners: which comes first, the generalist or the specialist? J R Soc Med [Internet]. 2014/02/13 ed. 2014 Mar;107(3): 99–102. https://pubmed.ncbi.nlm.nih.gov/24526462.
4. Stein H. Family medicine's identity: being generalists in a specialist culture? Ann Fam Med. 4(5):455–9.

5. Alam R, Cheraghi-Sohi S, Panagioti M, Esmail A, Campbell S, Panagopoulou E. Managing diagnostic uncertainty in primary care: a systematic critical review. BMC Fam Pract [Internet]. 2017 Aug 7;18(1):79. https://doi.org/10.1186/s12875-017-0650-0.

6. RCGP. MRCGP Exam Overview [Internet]. 2020. https://www.rcgp.org.uk/training-exams/mrcgp-exam-overview.aspx.

7. Nagendran M, Chen Y, Gordon AC. Real time self-rating of decision certainty by clinicians: a systematic review. Clin Med Lond Engl [Internet] 2019 Sep;19(5):369–74. https://pubmed.ncbi.nlm.nih.gov/31530683.

8. Balint M. The doctor, his patient and the illness. London: Churchill Livingstone; 1957.

9. Maslow AH. Theory of human motivation a. H. Maslow (1943) originally published in psychological review, 50, 370–396. Psychol Rev. 1943;50:370–96.

10. Berne E. Games people play. New York: Grove Press; 1964.

11. Byrne PS, Long EL. Doctors talking to patients : a study of the verbal behaviour of general practitioners consulting in their surgeries. London: RCGP; 1989.

12. Stott NC, Davis RH. The exceptional potential in each primary care consultation. J R Coll Gen Pract [Internet] 1979 Apr;29(201):201–5. https://pubmed.ncbi.nlm.nih.gov/448665.

13. Pendleton D. The new consultation: developing doctor-patient communication. Oxford: Oxford University Press; 2003.

14. Neighbour R. The inner consultation. MTP Press: Lancaster; 1987.

15. Foucault M. The birth of the clinic. Abingdon: Routledge; 2003.

16. Heath I. The mystery of general practice [Internet]. Nuffield Trust; 1985 [cited 2020 Dec 22]. Available from: Heath I. The mystery of general practice. Nuffield Provincial Hospitals Trust: 1995 http://www.nuffieldtrust.org.uk/sites/files/nuffield/publication/The_Mystery_of_General_Practice.pdf.

17. Bakhtin MM. The dialogic imagination: four essays. Austin: University of Texas Press; 1981.

18. Holland DC. Identity and agency in cultural worlds. Cambridge, MA: Harvard University Press; 1998.

19. Gramsci A, Hoare Q, Nowell-Smith G. Selections from the prison notebooks. London: Lawrence and Wishart; 1971.

20. Sandars J, Cook G. ABC of patient safety. Chichester: Wiley; 2009.

21. GPs asked to prescribe drugs and chase test results for secondary care inpatients. Pulse [Internet]. 2019 [cited 2020 Dec 22]. https://www.pulsetoday.co.uk/news/referrals/gps-asked-to-prescribe-drugs-and-chase-test-results-for-secondary-care-inpatients/.

22. Holland D, Lave J. History in person: enduring struggles, contentious practice, intimate identities. Santa Fe: School of American Research Press; 2001.

23. Lawson E. Debrief: the bleeding edge of neoliberalism. Br J Gen Pract [Internet]. 2019 Aug 1;69(685):390. http://bjgp.org/content/69/685/390.abstract.

24. Szymczak JE, Bosk CL. Training for efficiency: work, time, and systems-based practice in medical residency. J Health Soc Behav [Internet]. 2012 Aug 3 [cited 2020 Dec 23];53(3):344–358. https://doi.org/10.1177/0022146512451130.

25. McKee A. Learning organisations: the challenge of finding a safe space in a climate of accountability. Educ Prim Care [Internet]. 2017 Mar 4;28(2):72–4. https://doi.org/10.1080/14739879.2017.1283967.

26. Mayes C, Kerridge I, Habibi R, Lipworth W. Conflicts of interest in neoliberal times: perspectives of Australian medical students. Health Sociol Rev [Internet]. 2016 Sep 1;25(3):256–71. https://doi.org/10.1080/14461242.2016.1198713.

27. Black N. 'Liberating the NHS'-another attempt to implement market forces in English health care. N Engl J Med. 2010 Aug 25;363(12):1103–5.

28. Schrecker T. Neoliberalism and health: the linkages and the dangers. Sociol Compass [Internet]. 2016 Oct 1 [cited 2020 Dec 23];10(10):952–971. https://doi.org/10.1111/soc4.12408.

29. Fine B, Saad-Filho A. Thirteen things you need to know about neoliberalism. Crit Sociol [Internet]. 2016 Aug 19 [cited 2020 Dec 22];43(4–5):685–706. https://doi.org/10.1177/0896920516655387.

30. Liang R, Dornan T, Nestel D. Why do women leave surgical training? A qualitative and feminist study. The Lancet [Internet] 2019 Feb 9;393(10171):541–9. http://www.sciencedirect.com/science/article/pii/S0140673618326126.

31. Hill E, Solomon Y, Dornan T, Stalmeijer R. 'You become a man in a man's world': is there discursive space for women in surgery? Med Educ [Internet]. 2015 Dec 1 [cited 2020 Dec 23];49(12):1207–1218. https://doi.org/10.1111/medu.12818.

32. Chen MM, Yeo HL, Roman SA, Bell RH, Sosa JA. Life events during surgical residency have different effects on women and men over time. Surgery [Internet] 2013 Aug 1;154(2):162–70. http://www.sciencedirect.com/science/article/pii/S003960601300113X.

33. Mayorova T, Stevens F, Scherpbier A, van der Velden L, van der Zee J. Gender-related differences in general practice preferences: longitudinal evidence from the Netherlands 1982-2001. Health Policy. 2005;72(1):73–80.

34. Gale TCE, Lambe PJ, Roberts MJ. Factors associated with junior doctors' decisions to apply for general practice training programmes in the UK: secondary analysis of data from the UKMED project. BMC Med [Internet]. 2017 Dec 21;15(1):220. https://doi.org/10.1186/s12916-017-0982-6.

35. Alers M, van Leerdam L, Dielissen P, Lagro-Janssen A. Gendered specialities during medical education: a literature review. Perspect Med Educ [Internet]. 2014 Jun 1;3(3):163–78. https://doi.org/10.1007/s40037-014-0132-1.
36. Hill E, Vaughan S. The only girl in the room: how paradigmatic trajectories deter female students from surgical careers. Med Educ. 2013;47(6):547–56.

CHAPTER 5

Pedagogy, Policy and Practice

Abstract This chapter expands the sociocultural perspective of previous chapters to engage with specific concepts from Freire's critical pedagogy: specifically, casting GP training as a process of transformative learning which is deeply imbued with *troubled knowledge*. Translated into policy recommendations, a radical revision of training structures for GPs in the UK is suggested with a move away from the hegemonic assumptions of hospital-based training for community-based generalists.

Keywords GP training • NHS • Identity • Primary care • Educational policy • Postgraduate training

This chapter draws together the previous analyses and theoretical framework, and focuses on practical implications for practitioners and educators. Drawing on Paulo Freire's critical pedagogy, GP training is cast as a process of transformational learning imbued with *troubled knowledge*. Critically reviewing current policy and practice in the UK with regard to GP training, a radical shift is suggested away from hospital-based training for primary care doctors, with a total revision of training structures. The strengths and limitations of this approach are outlined with future directions for research in this essential part of medical training. A summary of key 'take-home' messages concludes the book.

CURRENT AND FUTURE CHALLENGES

The problematic structures of GP training both reflect and reify historical inequalities between primary and secondary care doctors. The contribution to healthcare made by GPs is large and growing, as a result of increased demand, fewer GPs and movement of services from secondary to primary care [1, 2]. In the UK, burnout was estimated to affect around a third of general practitioners even before the coronavirus pandemic of 2020 [3]. Improving the recruitment and retention of GPs has arguably never been of greater importance to care delivery [4].

The past, present and future of general practice in the NHS can be seen as an overarching narrative of change in response to crisis. Existing within a socialised healthcare system subject to neoliberal government agendas, care delivery in general practice is mediated by susceptibility to political influence [5–7]. The long-term future of NHS primary care looks uncertain from the viewpoint of 2020, where there are two major political events which may impact on training and practice: the on-going stressors of the pandemic and the UK's departure from the European Union with subsequent workforce impact [8–11].

Throughout the empirical narratives and theorisation of the primary care paradigm, an epistemology of medicine based on strong relational care could be seen. This offers an important corollary to industrialised neoliberal discourses of efficiency and accountability. The relational and humanistic care at the centre of general practice was a strong part of identifying as a GP for many of the trainees. Yet, could the very core of general practice's values be under threat? The trainees in the empirical studies were not followed beyond the original ethics remit, but they would have been expected to qualify as GPs in 2016 and, assuming they remained within the NHS, would be working as First 5 GPs at the time of writing in 2020. Newly qualified GPs in this position face new challenges and a clinical landscape shifting under their feet. The very aspects which are held most dear to GPs are those which are most susceptible to political discourse.

Already, the effects of the pandemic have been felt across primary care in a shift to 'total triage,' whereby all patients are screened by phone and much business done remotely. Longitudinal and relational care is being challenged and is at risk of falling prey to efficiency concerns [12]. This is a particular risk after the pandemic [13]. Meanwhile, fewer doctors are seeking a traditional GP partnership, as Maria figured for herself. The future of primary care may be one-off relationships, rather than longitudinal care, with knock-on effects on both patient care and education. Against this background of challenges to the very heart of the primary care paradigm, it is essential to give extra attention to how the socialisation of new GPs through education is achieved.

Conflicting Pedagogies

Critical pedagogy is a Marxist educational philosophy which originated with Brazilian educationalist Paulo Freire. Although operationalised in medical education in South America, critical pedagogy is little known in UK contexts. A critical pedagogy standpoint adopts an open-minded *problem-posing* approach, in which the social construction of knowledge is used to develop an awareness of inequality and the development of critical consciousness. This concept is particularly relevant to general practice work with deprived communities, as it eschews a biomedical model in recognition of sociocultural determinants of health.

For educationalists, critical pedagogy has a further application in recognising and addressing inherent inequalities perpetuated through training structures. The hospital component of GP training can be seen as an example of 'banking' knowledge, as was seen in Maria's narrative [14]. In terms of patient safety and experience, the question is how well-prepared GP trainees are for independent community practice, yet little to no effort is spent in the translation of knowledge for primary care use during secondary care placements. This task must then be undertaken mid-way through training on relocation to the community [15]. Workplace-based, situated learning is not given the same status as 'formal' training time in hospital, regardless of the quality or relevance of educational experience. It is included not for pedagogical reasons, but because of longstanding status assumptions and a pragmatic need for service delivery.

The identity threats encountered by GP trainees in hospital are a form of what is termed *troubled knowledge* [16]. This is a concept in critical pedagogy which pays attention to the present-day impact of previous difficult or traumatic experiences. The conflict engendered in trainees by negative messages about general practice in hospital must be resolved. This means either accepting or contesting the dominant hegemonic position of the secondary care paradigm, and its associated high-level discourses.

Given the sociocultural nature of education, it is an essential means of maintaining or contesting hegemony. To change negative positioning of primary care and the impact on GP identity, changes must be made to the structures of training.

Possibilities for Change

Increasing the Visibility of General Practice

For patients in the community, hospital admissions are a biographical disruption. Yet in medical education, the balance is reversed, with most medical education taking place in secondary care for the reasons outlined in Chap. 1. There is an inherent contradiction between patients' and doctors' experiences of healthcare [17].

One obvious step is increasing the visibility of the primary care paradigm at all levels of medical education. This entails not just increased curricular time, but an understanding from secondary care colleagues engaged in teaching of the nature of primary care. This would result in longer-term improvements to understanding and a reduction in paradigm conflict, with all medical students made aware of the key paradigm differences.

A second strategy is increasing the number of available F2 placements in general practice. Ideally, all foundation doctors should rotate through general practice at this stage of training. F2 placements are useful both for future hospital consultants, for whom it is likely to be their only experience working in primary care, but also for future GPs in increasing their awareness of the more challenging realities of the work.

GP Training Schemes

At the level of postgraduate GP training, there are both practical and ideological problems which should be addressed. There is a choice of more conservative or radical interventions here, with the feasibility of each likely to be influenced by political discourse and funding availability.

Arguably, most straightforward to address, requiring only extra training, is the lack of awareness of GP trainees' unique training needs amongst consultant supervisors. For example, it is well recognised that hospital educational supervisors and trainees both experience difficulties with training e-portfolios: supervisors with filling them in properly, and trainees with feeling that their forms are completed less well by hospital doctors than by GPs. The quality of feedback given by GP supervisors in Sabey and Harris' mixed methods study of hospital GP trainees was considered to be more worthwhile that that of consultant supervisors [15]. Issues like these may be amenable simply to training and quality control of supervision in hospital training environments from postgraduate deaneries.

A second strategy is to increase the primary care support available to GP trainees in hospital. It is evident that GP trainees in hospital occupy a marginal and at times uncomfortable position within hospital posts. These trainees are in particular need of support from general practice during this time. The current system of unprotected half-day monthly release is inadequate. As well as formal education, trainees would benefit from frequent contact with a GP mentor to help them 'debrief' and translate hospital experiences into primary care contexts. Making space within service provision for GP trainees to work within the community while they are based in hospital is an important compromise position short of radical adjustments to training.

More radical solutions are desirable, if less accessible, in pedagogical terms. Ultimately, hospital is unlikely to be the most appropriate learning environment for future GPs. Over the years, the hospital component of GP training has come under repeated scrutiny, as the need to provide sufficient numbers of junior doctors for NHS service provision competes with those doctors' individual developmental needs [18]. Evans et al. comment in their qualitative study that 'postgraduate general practice training in hospital-based posts was seen as poor quality, irrelevant and run as if it were of secondary importance to service commitments' [19]. Little has changed in this regard since this publication.

GP training in hospital needs to be urgently reviewed with a realignment towards educational priorities, rather than service ones. This is already the case in secondary care specialty training. Secondary care specialty trainees are not deployed to fill gaps in primary care delivery, and the opposite should cease to be true. Understanding the secondary care paradigm is essential for primary care trainees, but given the current structures of undergraduate and foundation training, the pedagogical argument for basing postgraduate GP trainees in hospital is dubious. Doctors in both primary and secondary care could gain knowledge of the others' work through 'in-reach' clinics and guided work experience.

Strengths, Limitations and Future Directions

Readers from a medical education background may come to this book with a diverse range of understandings of the world and of science. The approach taken throughout is based on a critical sociocultural approach to learning. This viewpoint sees knowledge as constructed and learning as a continuous process of adaptation to circumstances. Identity arises from daily practices and so sits close to learning.

This book is constructed around empirical narratives, which are then used to theorise the primary care paradigm and the nature of paradigm conflict. The sample used in the empirical analyses is small, in keeping with the philosophical approach to science. There has been no attempt here to recruit a statistically-significant sample, which would negate the depth of narrative and discourse analysis.

Because convenience and snowball sampling were used to recruit participants, there are obvious gaps. The predominantly female sample allows exploration of the intersection of gender with professional identity as it relates to them. It does not, however, permit extrapolation to male or non-binary GP trainees, groups for whom further research is recommended.

Similarly, there was an absence of racist influence or LGBTQI prejudice in the narratives, but these are important issues for GP training which deserve further investigation. Northern Ireland is undeniably more homogeneous than other areas of the UK, despite increasing diversity, and all the participants were white and from the island of Ireland. This situation is changing rapidly, however.

In theorising the primary and secondary care paradigms, the possibility is not excluded that further paradigms may exist (e.g. psychiatry).

It was stated in the first chapter that the analyses here are undertaken from an emic perspective. As the author and a practising GP, I was included within social understanding and language by the trainees acknowledging our joint membership of this 'club'. From a positivist biomedical perspective, this might be seen as bias. From a critical constructionist perspective, however, this relationship was a safe space which participants could use for sense-making through their narratives. Taking place in the research in the first place was a form of epistemological act for participants and a sense-making activity.

'Take Home' Points for Educators

Radical changes at a high policy level are subject to political discourse and may take long periods of time to engender change. In the meantime, on-the-ground changes can be achieved immediately and are likely to have a positive impact quickly. Hence, here are suggestions for directors of GP training programmes and educational supervisors (either hospital or GP):

- Recognising that medicine is not homogeneous, and that at least two distinct paradigms of care exist, is an important first step to increasing legitimacy and understanding of the primary care paradigm across the breadth of medicine.
- Understanding the nature of longstanding inequality and paradigm conflict as underpinning reduced status and negative messaging is a form of critical consciousness. By introducing these ideas and debriefing carefully with GP trainees based in hospitals, negative consequences may be minimised.
- Being critically conscious of medical education as a method of continuance of paradigm conflict, with implications far beyond unproblematic knowledge construction, is an important shift for educators.
- Embracing a critical awareness of these issues helps promote dialogue and cultural change in both education and the workplace, with benefits to patient care, professional performance and retention within the profession.

Conclusion

All education is political and potentially oppressive, but that same political quality gives it the possibility of being a vehicle for change. These chapters connect empirical narratives with other literature to theorise the subordinate position of general practice in the hierarchy of medicine and the conflicted position of GP trainees based in hospital.

Medicine is not homogeneous and medical training is not a smooth continuum, being rather a journey across a varied cultural landscape. The historically and socioculturally constructed inequality between primary and secondary care is reified and perpetuated by problematic systems of GP training, which place GPs in hospital contexts for half their training time. This paradigm conflict becomes part of the growing identity of GP trainees based in hospitals and is carried forward into community work. In this way, the basic inequality between primary and secondary care paradigms is perpetuated.

At policy level, radical changes to GP training could include a removal of the hospital component, with a greater focus on alternative ways of learning about the secondary care paradigm. At a pragmatic level, multiple small changes can improve this part of GP training in the shorter term. Improvements to structures of training have the ability to address ingrained power dynamics and paradigm conflict. These should be embraced to improve recruitment and retention to GP, with ultimate positive impact on patient care.

REFERENCES

1. Thompson M, Walter F. Increases in general practice workload in England. The Lancet [Internet]. 2016 Jun 4 [cited 2020 Dec 23];387(10035): 2270–2272. https://doi.org/10.1016/S0140-6736(16)00743-1.
2. Fisher RF, Croxson CH, Ashdown HF, Hobbs FR. GP views on strategies to cope with increasing workload: a qualitative interview study. Br J Gen Pract [Internet] 2017 Feb 1;67(655):e148. http://bjgp.org/content/67/655/e148.abstract.
3. Brown VT, Gregory S, Gray DP. The power of personal care: the value of the patient–GP consultation. Br J Gen Pract [Internet]. 2020 Dec 1;70(701):596. http://bjgp.org/content/70/701/596.abstract.
4. Marchand C, Peckham S. Addressing the crisis of GP recruitment and retention: a systematic review. Br J Gen Pract J R Coll Gen Pract [Internet]. 2017/03/13 ed. 2017 Apr;67(657):e227–e237. https://pubmed.ncbi.nlm.nih.gov/28289014.
5. Lawson E. Debrief: The bleeding edge of neoliberalism. Br J Gen Pract [Internet]. 2019 Aug 1;69(685):390. http://bjgp.org/content/69/685/390.abstract.
6. Abadía-Barrero CE, Bugbee M. Primary health Care for Universal Health Coverage? Contributions for a critical anthropological agenda. Med Anthropol [Internet]. 2019 Jul 4;38(5):427–35. https://doi.org/10.1080/0145974 0.2019.1620744.
7. Pollock A, Price D. Privatising primary care. Br J Gen Pract [Internet]. 2006 Aug 1;56(529):565. http://bjgp.org/content/56/529/565.abstract.
8. Health Service Journal, Geometric Results Inc. Brexit and the NHS workforce: a guide for healthcare leaders [internet]. HSJ. 2019; https://www.hsj.co.uk/workforce/brexit-and-the-nhs-workforce-a-guide-for-healthcare-leaders/7024658.article

9. Johnston JL, Hart N. Primary care education in the time of COVID: embodiment, identity and loss. Educ Prim Care [Internet]. 2020 Oct 28:1–4. https://doi.org/10.1080/14739879.2020.1837020

10. RCGP. Data shows GP workforce crisis still prevalent during pandemic, says RCGP [Internet]. [cited 2020 Dec 22]. https://www.rcgp.org.uk/about-us/news/2020/may/data-shows-gp-workforce-crisis-still-prevalent-during-pandemic-says-rcgp.aspx.

11. Dunlop C, Howe A, Li D, Allen LN. The coronavirus outbreak: the central role of primary care in emergency preparedness and response. BJGP Open [Internet] 2020 Apr 1;4(1):bjgpopen20X101041. http://bjgpopen.org/content/4/1/bjgpopen20X101041.abstract.

12. Park S, Abrams R, Wong G, Feder G, Mahtani KR, Barber J, et al. Reorganisation of general practice: be careful what you wish for. Br J Gen Pract [Internet]. 2019 Oct 1;69(687):517. http://bjgp.org/content/69/687/517.abstract.

13. Khan N, Jones D, Grice A, Alderson S, Bradley S, Carder P, et al. A brave new world: the new normal for general practice after the COVID-19 pandemic. BJGP Open [Internet]. 2020 Aug 1;4(3):bjgpopen20X101103. http://bjgpopen.org/content/4/3/bjgpopen20X101103.abstract.

14. Freire P. Pedagogy of the oppressed. New York: Herder and Herder; 1972.

15. Perera DP, Mohanna K. General practice is "different": a qualitative study of adaptation experiences of east Staffordshire general practice speciality trainees. Educ Prim Care [Internet]. 2020 Nov 27:1–9. https://doi.org/10.1080/14739879.2020.1836520

16. Zembylas M. Critical pedagogy and emotion: working through 'troubled knowledge' in posttraumatic contexts. Crit Stud Educ [Internet]. 2013 Jun 1;54(2):176–89. https://doi.org/10.1080/17508487.2012.743468.

17. Lee SWW, Clement N, Tang N, Atiomo W. The current provision of community-based teaching in UK medical schools: an online survey and systematic review. BMJ Open [Internet] 2014 Dec 1;4(12):e005696. http://bmjopen.bmj.com/content/4/12/e005696.abstract.

18. Capewell S, Stewart K, Bowie P, Kelly M. Trainees' experiences of a four – year programme for specialty training in general practice. Educ Prim Care. 2014;25:18–25.

19. Evans J, Lambert T, Goldacre M. GP recruitment and retention: a qualitative analysis of doctors' comments about training for and working in general practice. Occas Pap R Coll Gen Pract. 83:1–33.